Incorporating Natural Products into the Human Diet

INCORPORATING NATURAL PRODUCTS INTO THE HUMAN DIET

Edited by:

Laghulkar Anita Marotirao

Delve
PUBLISHING

www.delvepublishing.com

Incorporating Natural Products into the Human Diet

Laghulkar Anita Marotirao

Delve Publishing
224 Shoreacres Road
Burlington, ON L7L 2H2
Canada
www.delvepublishing.com
Email: orders@arclereducation.com

ISBN: 978-1-77469-481-7 (Hardcover)

ABOUT THE EDITOR

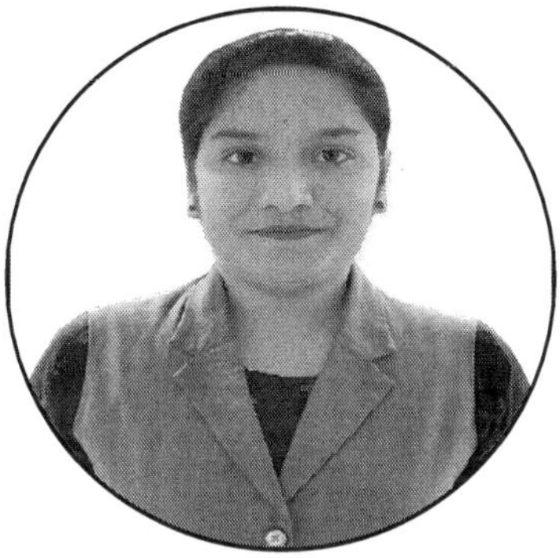

Miss Anita Laghulkar is presently serving as Assistant professor, Department of Food Chemistry and Nutrition, College of Food Technology Naigaon (Bz) Nanded, Maharashtra affiliated by Vasantrao Naik Marathwada Krishi Vidyapith, Parbhani. She obtained her B.Tech (Food Technology) in 2016 from College of Food Technology Naigaon & M.Tech (Food process Technology) in 2018 from Maharashtra Institute of Technology Aurangabad, Maharashtra. She started her career as Assistant professor in 2018. Her M.Tech specialization in reduction of acrylamide compound from processed Food. She has published 2 research paper in international journal. She has participated in many National and international symposiums and state seminar.

TABLE OF CONTENTS

LIST OF FIGURES

ABSTRACT

This volume sums up existing evidence on the effect of natural food on human health. It examines organic versus traditional food production in regards to human health and examines the possible effect of natural management activities universally. Natural food consumption might lessen the risk of contracting allergic illnesses and obesity, however, the evidence isn't definitive due to possible residual confounding, as buyers of natural food will quite often have better lifestyles generally speaking. In any case, animal tests propose that products made from natural or traditional foods impact in various ways on development and improvement. In organic farming, the utilization of pesticides is limited, while deposits in regular foods grown from the ground form the primary source of human pesticide risks. Epidemiological research has detailed the negative impacts of specific pesticides on youngsters' cognitive capacity at existing degrees of risk, however, these data have up until this point not been applied in conventional risk evaluations of individual pesticides. Contrasts in the structure between natural and traditional harvests are limited, for example, a higher amount of phenolic compounds in natural leafy foods, and a reasonably reduced amount of cadmium in natural grain crops. Organic dairy items, and some meats, additionally have a higher ratio of omega-3 fatty acids contrasted with traditional food products.

PREFACE

Nutrient-packed food varieties are low in sodium, sugar, starches, and bad fats. They contain many vitamins and minerals and scarcely any calories. The body requires vitamins and minerals, called micronutrients. They feed the body and assist with keeping one healthy. This volume proposes that supplements can lessen the risk of terminal infections. Consuming nutritious food guarantees the body can assimilate them appropriately. Food sources that are high in calories and low in micronutrients likewise contain added sugar, sodium (salt), and trans-fats. This kind of diet adds to weight gain. It can increase the chances of medical problems, like coronary illness and type 2 diabetes. Most nutrient-dense foods varieties are unpopular since they aren't often sweet, for example, broccoli.

During flu seasons, people frequently look for unique food sources or nutrient supplements that are understood to boost immunity. L-ascorbic acid and food varieties such as citrus products, chicken soup, and honey tea are well-known models. However, the structure of our immune system is complicated and impacted by an optimal equilibrium of many variables, not just diet, and particularly not by any particular food or vitamin. Nonetheless, a balanced diet comprising of the scope of nutrients and minerals, together with healthy life factors like satisfactory rest and exercise and low pressure, most really takes action to combat contamination and illness. Consistently, people are at risk of unsafe organisms, everything being equal. The body immunity, a system of complex stages and body pathways safeguards against harmful microorganisms as well as specific infections. It distinguishes unfamiliar invaders like microscopic organisms, viruses, and parasites and takes prompt action.

The volume mentions that people have two kinds of immunity: adaptive and innate. The latter is a first-line safeguard from microorganisms that attempt to enter the body, accomplished through defensive barriers. These obstacles include skin that prevents microorganisms, bodily fluid that traps microbes, stomach acid that obliterates microbes, chemicals in our perspiration and tears that assist with fighting against bacterial mixtures, and defensive cells that prevent bad cells from entering the body.

Adaptive immunity is a system that determines how to distinguish a microbe. It is directed by cells and organs in the body like the spleen, thymus, bone marrow, and lymph nodes. Whenever an unfamiliar substance enters the body, these cells and organs make antibodies and lead to the augmentation of safe cells counting various kinds of white platelets, which are well defined as unsafe substances that affect the body. The safe system then adjusts by recalling the unfamiliar substance so that assuming harmful substances are present, these antibodies and cells will considerably more effectively destroy it. The volume further mentions different circumstances that might set off an immune reaction, for example, antigens which are substances that the body considers unfamiliar and unsafe, and may set off safety measures. Allergens are one kind of antigen and incorporate grass pollen, dust, food parts, or pet hair. Antigens can cause allergic reactions in which too many white cells are produced by the body.

CHAPTER 1

HUMAN NUTRITION

CONTENTS

The human body may be thought of as an engine that creates energy from the food we eat. This energy performs a variety of purposes, including muscular and secretory work, as well as the preservation of the body's structure and functioning. To maintain a healthy body temperature, the abilities to create heat and manage heat loss must be combined. The human body, unlike other engines, is continually disintegrating, catabolizing, and recreating or analyzing its component components. Foods supply the nutrients and energy required for the chemical reactions required for the production of new materials (Yousuf et al., 2021)

Proper nutrition is essential for human life, health, and development. Proper nutrition is vital for survival, physical growth, mental development, performance and productivity, health, and well-being at all stages of life, including birth, infancy, youth, adolescence, and old age.

It is necessary for both personal and national development. Everyone should have the chance to acquire and maintain the highest possible health throughout their lives, according to WHO's fundamental aim of "health for all. Amid poverty, misery, and malnutrition, this is incomprehensible

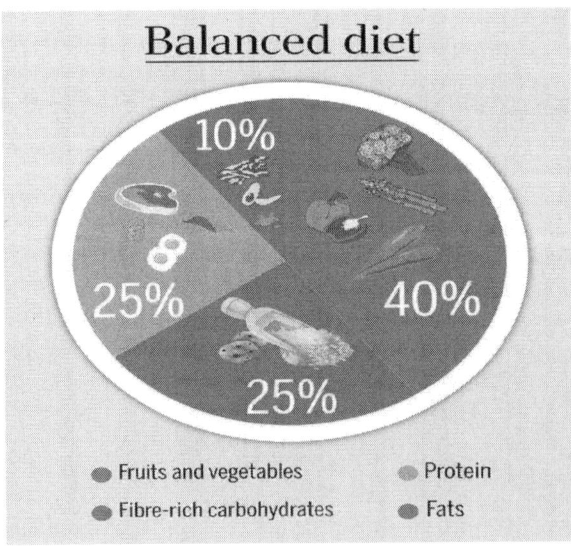

Figure 1.1: A balanced diet should contain fats, protein, carbs, and vegetables.

It is the study of food and nutrient availability and utilization in people to ensure one's own life, good health, and ability to grow and develop appropriately. Human nutrition covers a wide range of topics, from biology and metabolic nutrition to whole-body and clinical nutrition, as well as the massive public health nutrition challenges confronting national nutrition programs and the global prevention, control, and eradication of malnutrition and nutritional diseases. It is a vast subject. Because of its fundamental importance for human health and development, the WHO has consistently highlighted nutrition as a crucial component of its mandate from its foundation in 1948.

The World Health Organization (WHO) focuses on critical areas such as basic nutritional research, nutrition therapy from infancy to old age, and, most significantly, nutrition policies and programs for long-term development at all levels (Walker *et al.,* 2015). A range of factors impacts nutritional well-being, including diet, health, and the surrounding environment. Each dietary component has a direct influence on human health in the subject of human nutrition.

Individual life events and heredity determine how much food a person consumes concerning their body composition. A healthy lean man's physique is composed of more water than fat, more protein than minerals, and more carbohydrate than minerals. For good measure, there are trace amounts of other vitamins and minerals scattered throughout. It is believed that women have around 22 percent of their total body weight (in a healthy lean woman), whereas males have approximately 17 percent.

To maintain homeostasis, or dynamic balance, the body's various compartments, which include lean body mass, body fat, and body water, continually adjust to changes in the internal and external environment. Catabolism and anabolism are the mechanisms through which the tissues of the body are constantly destroyed and regenerated at various rates. Red blood cells last for 120 days, whereas connective tissue regenerates over time and digestive tract epithelial cells are replaced every three to four days.

A direct inspection can be used to calculate the proportion of body fat, although this approach is unreliable. Indirect ways include underwater weighing, potassium measurement in the entire body, and dual-energy X-ray absorptiometry. DXA may be used to calculate body fat. Despite their practicality and lower accuracy, methods such as anthropometry — which uses skinfold calipers to measure subcutaneous fat at various locations — bioelectrical impedance — which measures resistance to a low-intensity electrical current — and near-infrared interactants — which measures fat and protein interaction by shining an infrared light on the biceps — are more commonly used. Only cadavers can be used to directly measure the body's various compartments (Vanbergen & Initiative, 2013).

People's dietary demands change as they age, and the makeup of their bodies changes throughout time. This is especially true throughout life's critical years, such as puberty, pregnancy, and nursing. Maintaining an active lifestyle can assist people to avoid the loss of lean tissue and rise in body fat that occurs as they age.

For example, the process by which food components generate energy or are converted into human tissues is only the beginning of this trip, which leads to illnesses caused by a shortage or excess of critical nutrients, such as malnutrition. Dietary components are currently being examined for their involvement in the development of chronic degenerative disorders such as coronary heart disease, cancer, and dental caries.

The food we eat influences a wide range of human processes, including prenatal health and development and the ability to resist sickness. As nutritional science and molecular biology collide, dietary components and the vast variety of human physiological responses are increasingly being explored at the cellular level. Furthermore, nutrition considers why people eat the foods they do, even if they are harmful to their health.

Eating habits are studied by the social sciences of psychology, anthropology, sociology, and economics. Dietetics or community nutrition refers to the use of nutritional knowledge to promote people's health and well-being. Dietitians counsel people on how to improve their health via dietary modifications and can also cure illnesses. Many people work in the manufacture, preparation, and distribution of meals that encourage these activities (Turner & Thompson, 2013).

To various people, a healthy diet entails different things. Parents, teachers, and physicians who are concerned about their children's growth and development are concerned about their children's nutrition. For the wealthy, nutrition science has shifted its focus to achieving optimal health and 'delaying' chronic degenerative disorders with intricate etiologies such as obesity, cardiovascular disease, cancer, and diabetes.

To grow, all living creatures require a particular quantity of nutrients, which are referred to as "essential nutrients." There can be no life if there is no water. By the late nineteenth century, several critical amino acids and inorganic elements, including calcium, potassium, iodine, and iron, had been found in proteins.

The cornerstones of nutritional well-being are good health and proper nutrition. To guarantee optimum nutrition, infectious illness prevention and treatment are critical. If immediate action is to be taken, everyone must have access to proper health care services. Immunization, early detection and treatment of infectious diseases such as tuberculosis, health, and nutrition education, and growth monitoring are just a few examples (Tang *et al.*, 2020).

How many grams of each meal and beverage do individuals consume daily, and how frequently? The individual's reaction will never be accurate unless they are isolated in a separate research center and constantly monitored. People may not notice or recall the particular description of their meals, especially when served on mixed plates, making it difficult to obtain objective information on calorie consumption. When asked to keep track of their food intake, people's diets may change. It is difficult to create a profile of a person's usual diet since they do not consume the same foods every day. Several strategies were employed.

A simple computation divides the total amount of food produced and sold by the estimated population of the nation. This is how food vanishes or approaches consumption. There's no question that some stuff is discarded, while others are consumed by visitors and their dogs.

This data collection makes it easy to track national trends and determine if consumers consume too much or too little of a certain food item. The alternate technique records people's exact meals as well as the quantity consumed. These approaches frequently rely on patients' recollections or oblige them to keep a journal of everything they ingest for a set period.

1.1 ESSENTIAL NUTRIENTS AND THEIR FUNCTIONS

Carbohydrates, fats and oils, protein, vitamins, minerals, and water are all part of the diet. Every day, around 500 grams (little more than one pound) of carbohydrates, fats, and proteins are ingested into the diet. These macronutrients supply the basic ingredients for tissue development and repair, as well as the energy for the body's numerous physiological and metabolic processes. Micronutrients such as vitamins (300 milligrams per day) and minerals (1,000 milligrams per day) do not generate energy but rather support metabolic processes throughout the body (20 grams per day). Water is the final nutritional category to address since it is the carrier for all of the body's metabolic operations. In most circumstances, this label is given to nutrients that must be obtained via food to be termed "essential."

1.1.1 Carbohydrates

Carbohydrates, which are made up of carbon, hydrogen, and oxygen, provide the majority of the body's energy and provide 4 kcal per gram. Because most carbs include hydrogen and oxygen in a 2:1 ratio, carbon is referred to as "carbohydrate," while water is referred to as "hydrate."

Carbohydrates provide the majority of the energy for the brain. You cannot operate effectively until you consume carbs. Carbohydrates can be found in starchy vegetables, sweets, and fruits. You should try to consume at least half of your grain diet like whole grains. Consuming fiber-rich whole grains and fruit makes it simpler to maintain a healthy blood sugar level. Sugars are the most basic carbohydrates, and they may be found in a variety of foods, but they can also nourish bacteria in the mouth, which can lead to tooth decay. The two types of sugars found in the diet are monosaccharides and disaccharides (Stintzing & Carle, 2004). Energy is provided by disaccharides such as sucrose, lactose, and maltose, as well as monosaccharides such as glucose, fructose, and galactose. Beans and other legumes have an oligosaccharide that humans are unable to break down, which contributes to their gas-inducing properties. Polysaccharides are lengthy chains of glucose molecules utilized to store more complex carbohydrate compounds. Starch, the most abundant polysaccharide in the human diet, is made up of either straight (amylose) or primarily branched glucose chains (amylopectin). The majority of polysaccharides in the human diet are starches. It is found in grains, beans, potatoes, and several other plants. Amylopectin, the most prevalent kind, is a mix of straight and branched glucose chains. The digestible polysaccharides known as dietary fiber, which are abundant in plant-based diets, are deficient in vegetables and fruits, legumes, seeds, and nuts.

All complex carbohydrates must first be reduced to simple sugars to be broken down into monosaccharides. The majority of absorption occurs in the small intestine and is carried out by enzymes. Specialist enzymes, such as lactase, which breaks down lactose into its monosaccharides, glucose, and galactose, break down disaccharides into monosaccharides. Lactase activity drops in a large percentage of the world's population between infancy and adolescence, resulting in an inability to digest lactose correctly. Lactose intolerance develops when a person consumes too much lactose, and it is passed down through the family.

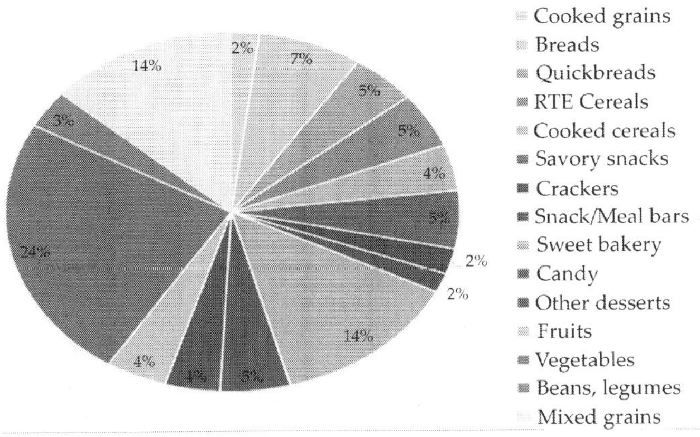

Figure 1.2: Carbohydrate food examples.

(Source: Drewnowski A., Maillot M., et al., 2022)

1.1.2 Protein

Protein, in addition to being the most significant structural component of cells, is also involved in the formation and mending of human tissues. When protein is broken down into its constituent amino acids, amino acids are generated. Nine of the twenty amino acids are considered "essential amino acids" since the body is unable to synthesize them on its own and must thus be obtained from food. Nitrogen is part of the amino chemical group NH2, and sulfur may be present in proteins, polysaccharides, and lipids under certain circumstances. Proteins are crucial components of the human body because they act as biochemical catalysts and gene regulators. Protein is the building block of muscles, bones, internal organs, skin, nails, and hair, as well as water. Proteins such as hemoglobin can be found in cell membranes and blood. Proteins that accelerate chemical processes in the body include enzymes, antibodies, collagen in connective tissue, and other hormones such as insulin (Shipp & Abdel-Aal, 2010).

Proteins are continually broken down and resynthesized to fulfill the body's demands to maintain and repair tissues. Protein intake from meals and protein losses through the kidneys, feces, and skin maintain a dynamic balance between tissue proteins and blood proteins. Adults in excellent health should make the required modifications to balance their protein losses and intakes. The body maintains a positive nitrogen balance during periods of fast development, pregnancy, and lactation, or recovery from disease or tiredness; the contrary is true during times of sluggish development, pregnancy, lactation, or recovery from illness or exhaustion. Lean protein meals, such as low-fat meat, dairy, beans, or eggs, should account for 10% to 35% of your daily calorie consumption.

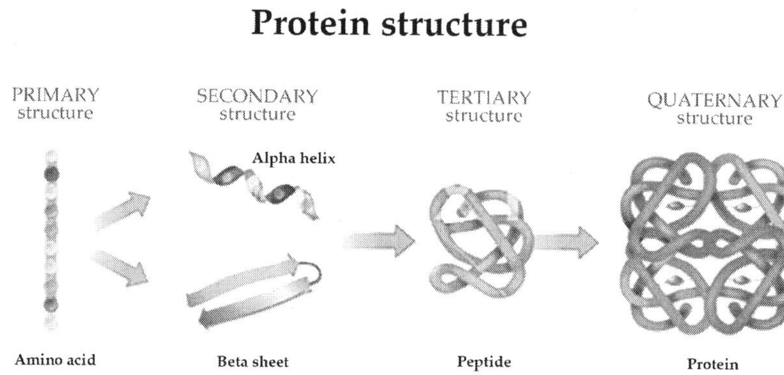

Figure 1.3: Protein structure.

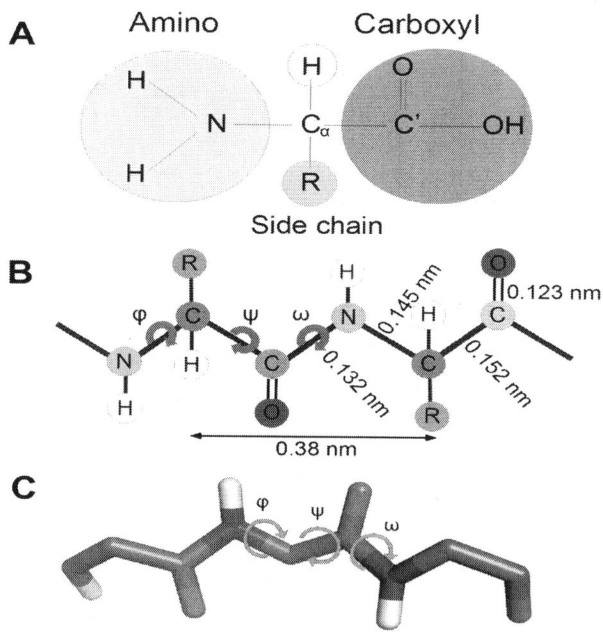

Figure 1.4: Protein amino acid structure.

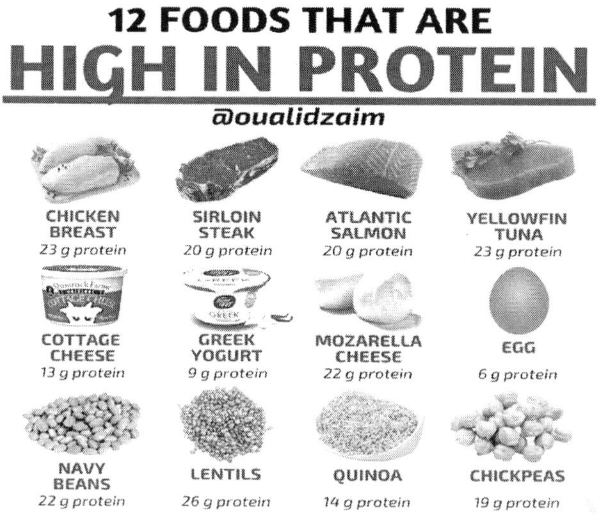
12 FOODS THAT ARE
HIGH IN PROTEIN
@oualidzaim
CHICKEN BREAST
23 g protein
SIRLOIN STEAK
20 g protein
ATLANTIC SALMON
20 g protein
YELLOWFIN TUNA
23 g protein
COTTAGE CHEESE
13 g protein
GREEK YOGURT
9 g protein
MOZARELLA CHEESE
22 g protein
EGG
6 g protein
NAVY BEANS
22 g protein
LENTILS
26 g protein
QUINOA
14 g protein
CHICKPEAS
19 g protein

Figure 1.5: Examples of protein foods.

1.2 LIPIDS IS THE NAME GIVEN TO THIS FORM OF FAT

Carbon, hydrogen, and oxygen are all present in lipids, although in a slightly different order than in carbohydrates. The separation of an oil-and-vinegar salad dressing demonstrated that lipids are soluble in organic solvents such as acetone or ether but not in water. Triglycerides, fats, oils, phospholipids, and sterols such as cholesterol are all nutritionally essential lipids. Lipids in food aid in the transportation and absorption of fat-soluble vitamins A, D, E, and K in the small intestine. In addition to satiety-inducing chemicals, many meals have a sensory appeal, as well as a nice flavor and texture, which make eating a meal a happy experience (Sharma et al., 2021). Fats have a larger energy level in the diet than carbs, with nine kcal per gram. Adipose tissue, also known as fatty tissue, is found in the body's fat depots and acts as an energy source as well as an insulator and cushion for the organs.

When fat is ingested, fat-soluble vitamins such as A, D, E, and K are better absorbed. Fat should account for between 20% and 35% of your daily calorie intake. Salmon, walnuts, and vegetable oils rich in omega-3 fatty acids are all good substitutes. Taking omega-3 fatty acids has several health advantages. Consume nuts, seeds, and avocado instead of saturated fats found in full-fat dairy products such as milk and cheese.

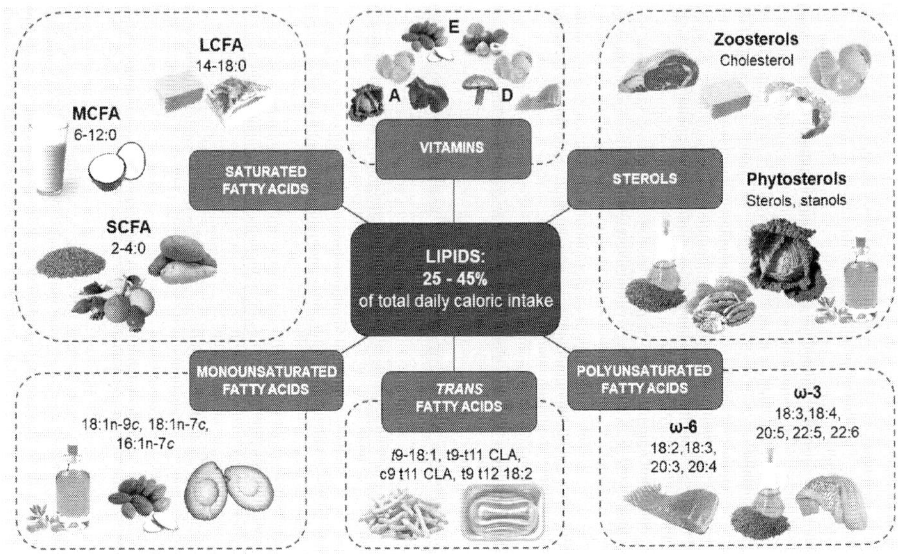

Figure 1.6: Examples of food that contain fats.

(Source: Papotti B, Escolà-Gil JC et, al.,2021)

1.3 VITAMINS AND MINERALS ARE NECESSARY FOR OPTIMAL HEALTH

All living things require vitamins, which are organic substances found in little amounts in food. To a limited extent, humans can synthesize several vitamins. Niacin is derived from the amino acid tryptophan; vitamin K is produced by bacteria in our intestines; and biotin, vitamin K, and vitamin D are all produced by our bodies. Food, on the other hand, provides vitamins to the human body.

Although many fruits and vegetables include vitamin C and beta-carotene, water provides the majority of their calories and protein. While fresh veggies are a rich source of vitamin C, cooked vegetables aren't so much. Vitamin A levels are very high in dark-green leafy vegetables. Vegetables also contain calcium and iron, which are difficult to absorb. Sugar is abundant in fruits and vegetables such as apples, oranges, and berries. Bananas are high in potassium. Constipation may be avoided by consuming lots of fiber, which is found in many fruits and vegetables (Acosta-Estrada *et al.*, 2021).

A vitamin deficiency illness develops when the body is deficient in or unable to utilize a specific vitamin. If addressed early on, the signs and symptoms of a vitamin deficiency can be reversed. Vitamin amounts are estimated in milligrams and micrograms at each meal, as well as the total quantity required for the year.

Macronutrients provide energy and raw materials for tissue synthesis in the body, whereas vitamins do not. They play an important part in energy generation, as well as metabolic and physiologic functions. Furthermore, vitamin A is necessary for optimal immune system function, epithelial cellular integrity, and embryonic growth and development. Folate, often known as folic acid, is a B vitamin that acts as a coenzyme to help prevent birth abnormalities during the first trimester of pregnancy. Vitamin C is an antioxidant that safeguards the body against free radicals. This chemical also aids in the formation of connective tissue. Vitamin D, a hormone, regulates calcium and phosphorus levels in the body as well as bone metabolism. Vitamin E defends lipid systems against free radical damage, whereas vitamin K aids in blood clotting. Both vitamin E and vitamin K are antioxidants. A deficiency in one vitamin can impair the functioning of another.

Each of the thirteen vitamins required by humans may be grouped into two groups of three based on their solubility. Fat-soluble vitamins A, D, E, and K may be dissolved using nonpolar solvents. Calcitriol, the vitamin D hormone, is still classified as a vitamin even though it now works as a hormone. Vitamin C and the B-complex vitamins are among the nine water-soluble vitamins. Among these are vitamins B6 and B12, folic acid, pantothenic acid, and biotin. Chlorophyll is a vitamin-like food component that the human body can make on its own (Shockley & Dossey, 2014). Although its importance in the human diet throughout life has not been proven, preterm newborns and people with certain medical problems may require choline in their diets.

Different environmental and chemical factors make many vitamins more or less prone to degradation. Thiamin, for example, is susceptible to prolonged heating; riboflavin, to UV or fluorescent light; and vitamin C, to oxidation in the presence of air. Cooking degrades water-soluble vitamins faster than fat-soluble vitamins.

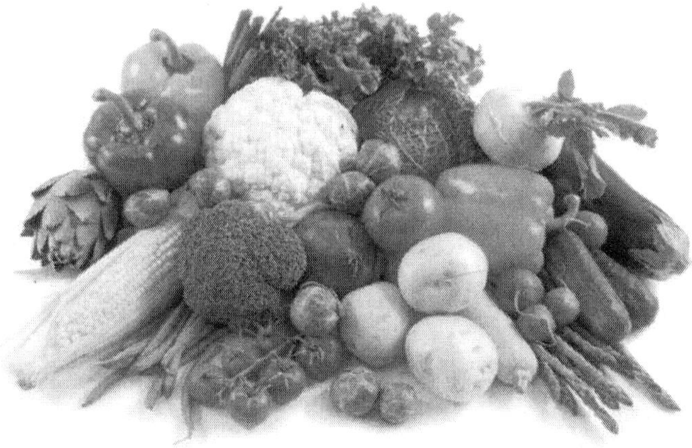

Figure 1.7: Examples of food that have vitamins.

Source: https://cdn.britannica.com/93/157193-004-943016F7.jpg

Vitamin solubility influences the body's capacity to absorb, transport, store, and eliminate vitamins, as does vitamin location in food. All water-soluble vitamins, except for vitamin B12, are generated by plants and may be found in both plant and animal diets. Vegans and strict vegetarians who forgo all animal foods may suffer from vitamin B12 insufficiency. Fat-soluble vitamins, on the other hand, are found in meals in the body with fats and oils and normally require protein carriers to bridge the body's water-filled compartments, which is why they are termed fat-soluble vitamins.

Water-soluble vitamins, except for vitamin B12, cannot be stored in the body and must thus be ingested regularly. Even water-soluble vitamins, such as vitamin B6, can be detrimental if consumed in large quantities; vitamin B6 is particularly prominent in this regard. Fat-soluble vitamins do not need to be ingested every day since they are stored in the liver and fatty tissue and may thus be consumed at levels that fulfill the body's demands over long periods. However, due to the vitamins' propensity to store energy, taking too high a dose may result in dangerous side effects. Toxic doses of vitamins A and D are extremely hazardous. In rare cases, pharmacological "megadoses" of several vitamins have been demonstrated to be useful (Saberi et al., 2017). Vitamin A compounds are used in pharmaceuticals to treat acne and other skin disorders, as well as wrinkles, and vitamin D is used to cure psoriasis. Over supplementation with vitamins and other nutrients, on the other hand, is not recommended except under medical supervision.

Vitamin C can only play its function via promoting the creation of collagen, which is required for the structural integrity of blood vessels, bones, and ligaments. Citrus fruits, strawberries, and peppers, which are all high in vitamin C, may be found. The vitamin folate, which may be found in several foods, helps to prevent birth defects. Pregnant women and women attempting to conceive should take folic acid, a synthetic form of folate. Calcium homeostasis can only be maintained by vitamin D. Many foods contain it, and the sun naturally creates it.

1.4 MINERALS

In contrast to the complex organic compounds (carbohydrates, lipids, proteins, and vitamins) outlined above, a mineral is a simple inorganic element that is neither digested nor used for energy. Elements account for 4 percent to 6 percent of a person's weight on average, with calcium and phosphorus accounting for half and the remainder coming from nutrition. Minerals are used in metabolism in a variety of ways, including as electrolytes that regulate the flow of water into and out of cells, as components of enzyme systems, and as components of a wide variety of organic compounds (Rochfort, 2005). Minerals are classified into two types: those that are naturally present in the organism and those that the organism requires for health and well-being. The majority of people require at least 100 mg of these macrominerals, which comprise calcium, phosphorus, magnesium, sulfur, and sodium chloride, every day. As part of the vitamin B12 molecule, a variety of trace elements are required in modest amounts of 15 mg or less per day. Iron, zinc, copper, manganese, iodine, selenium, fluoride, molybdenum, chromium, and cobalt are among the trace elements. Despite the lack of nutritional value, it is considered a healthy dinner due to fluoride's role in preventing dental cavities.

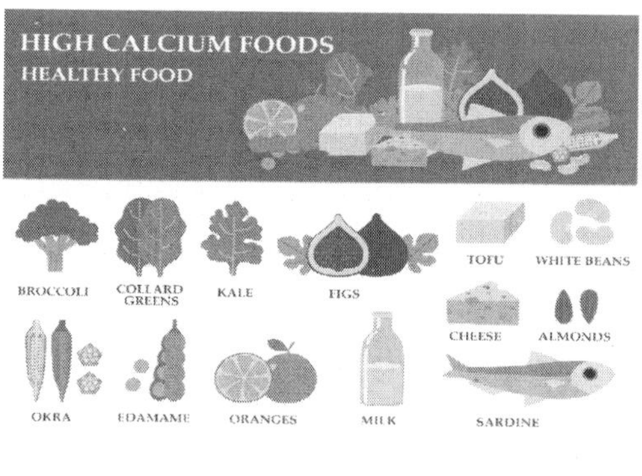

Figure 1.8: Some high calcium foods include sardine, milk, kale, tofu, and figs.

Arsenic, a mineral present in extremely low amounts in food and human tissue, is an example of an ultra-trace element (micrograms per day). Even though these and other ultra-trace elements are employed in animal tests, we still don't know what role they play in human tissues or how significant they are to human health.

Minerals are required for many body activities, including muscular contraction, nerve transmission, blood coagulation, and blood pressure and growth regulation. Except for sulfur, sodium, potassium, magnesium, and calcium exist as positive ions or cations, and chloride and phosphates as negative ions or anions, throughout the body. Mineral salts aid in the regulation of fluid, osmotic pressure, and acid-base balance in physiological fluids.

Sodium regulates the quantity of fluid outside the cells, which is necessary for cell activity. Keep your daily consumption to a maximum of 2,400 milligrams. Potassium reduces the formation of hypertension when salt consumption is increased by managing fluid content both within and outside cells. Bananas, potatoes, and tomatoes are potassium-rich foods. Calcium is required for the development and maintenance of bones and teeth. Every day, three servings of calcium-rich foods such as milk, low-fat cheese, and yogurt are recommended (Ribeiro *et al.*, 2019).

The mineral content of meals is influenced by growth factors such as soil and water composition, as well as how food is digested. Mineral ash from a full meal may be burnt without affecting the mineral composition. Minerals leached from spent cooking water, on the other hand, may be lost.

A variety of variables impact mineral absorption and availability in the body. Minerals are more easily absorbed in animal-based diets than in plant-based diets. Fiber and other absorption obstacles are present in the latter. The interaction of physic acid, which is typically present in wheat and legumes, with phytic acid can generate insoluble and indigestible minerals. The high content of oxalic acid in spinach limits calcium absorption by binding to calcium and preventing it from being absorbed by the body. Iron supplementation can limit zinc absorption, whereas an excess of zinc can impair copper absorption. Non-human iron can be absorbed with sufficient vitamin C, whereas calcium can be absorbed with sufficient vitamin D. Mineral absorption is also regulated by the mineral's present physiological need.

Minerals, unlike many vitamins, have a smaller spectrum of potential adverse effects. Minerals, even in little amounts, can be dangerous if used in more than authorized doses. This is especially true for trace elements found in significant quantities, such as iron and copper. Accidental iron supplementation is the leading cause of death in children under the age of five.

1.5 WATER

Despite its lack of official classification as a nutrient, water, or H2O, is the most important of all nutrients. Humans can survive for weeks without food, but just a few days without water before they die. A multitude of biochemical events occurs in the body as metabolism develops, including the transport of nutrients and waste products. Water not only regulates body temperature, blood pressure, and volume, but it also influences the form of big molecules and the tensile strength of human tissues. It acts as a protective cushion and solvent in the eyelids, spinal fluid, and amniotic fluid (Reis *et al.*, 2017). The quantity of water that enters and exits cells may be controlled by altering the electrolyte contents at each end of the cell membrane. Intracellular electrolytes include potassium, magnesium, phosphate, and sulfate, whereas external electrolytes include sodium and chloride.

A healthy adult's body weight is made up of around half to three-quarters water, but this figure skyrockets in youngsters. Because lean tissue stores around three-quarters of its weight in water and fatty tissue contains approximately one-fifth of its weight in water, body composition, particularly the amount of fat, influences the body water percentage. To put it another way, men have more lean tissue than women, which means they have more water in their bodies. Water content is high in various foods, including fruits and vegetables, which can contain up to 95 percent of their whole weight in water.

Water is produced by the body as a consequence of the metabolic activities that occur within it. Each day, the elimination of urine, water vapor from the lungs, perspiration loss from the skin, and feces exchange around 2.5 liters of water (2.6 quarts). There is no general advice for daily water intake because the amount of water required varies on several factors such as climate, degree of exercise, meal composition, and so on. Adults, on the other hand, require at least 8 glasses of water each day from all sources. Thirst is not a good indicator of dehydration since it arises before the body is ordered to restore fluids. Water consumption should be promoted throughout the day, even in hot climates, during vigorous physical exercise, or in dehydrating conditions such as an airline ride.

Water hydrates and nourishes the body's cells. Water also aids in the removal of waste from the body. Soup, watermelon, and other high-moisture meals contain water, which helps you achieve your daily water need. Adults should drink between 2 and 3 liters of water every day, depending on their weight (Raes et al., 2004).

There are several nutrients, such as vitamins and minerals. Citrus, berries, tropical, drupes, pomes, and melons are only six of the numerous vitamin and mineral-rich fruits.

Citrus fruits, which include grapefruit, oranges, tangerines, and lemons, are high in vitamin C, potassium, and folate. Vitamin C strengthens the immune system and hence aids collagen formation. Vitamins B12 and folate are essential for the proper functioning of the heart and cells, respectively, while potassium aids in the maintenance of normal blood pressure. The term "berry" refers to a wide range of fruits and vegetables that resemble berries. Among these are antioxidants and phytonutrients, both of which can reduce inflammation.

Tropical fruits include papaya, kiwi, and pineapple, among others. These fruits provide a variety of nutrients that can benefit bone health, blood sugar management, thyroid function, and nervous system function. Several types of drupe fruits fit under this group. Other nutrients include vitamin C, potassium, and beta carotene. Beta carotene, which is present in many fruits and vegetables, benefits both the eyes and the immune system. several fruits, including apples and pears, vitamin C, and potassium. Melon, including watermelon, cantaloupe, honeydew, and casaba, is high in vitamin C.

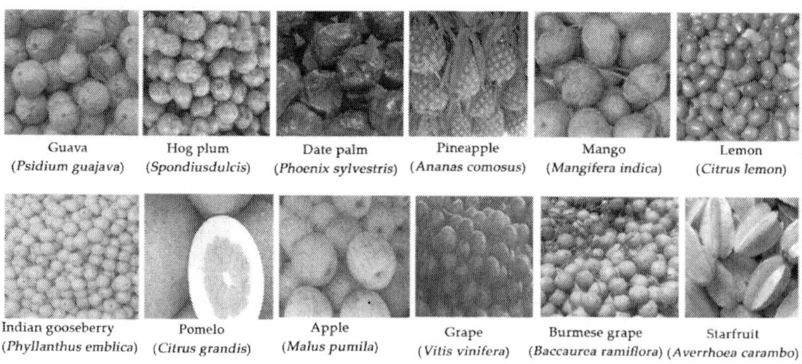

Figure 1.9: Fruits.

(Source: Rahman MM, Azad MOK, et, al., 2021)

1.6 FIBER

Smoothies made from mixed fruits can help you meet your daily fiber requirements, which vary from 25 to 38 grams for women and men, respectively. Blackberries, pears, and apples all include five to seven grams of fiber per serving, which is more than the two to four grams found in most fruits. By delaying digestion, the insoluble fiber in fruits may help regulate blood sugar and cholesterol levels (Proksch *et al.,* 2003).

1.7 SMOOTHIE'S FOUNDATION

You may use whatever you choose as the foundation for your smoothie. To boost the amount of fruit, add water, milk, soy milk, or yogurt. If you want something with fewer calories, you may use water, low-fat milk, or low-fat yogurt. Water's role as a body fluid allows for nutritional digestion and absorption. Low-fat dairy products provide calcium and vitamin D, both of which are essential for strong bones.

1.8 NUTRIENTS THAT CANNOT BE MANUFACTURED BY THE HUMAN BODY

Your body produces a wide range of non-essential nutrients that it needs to function. Essential nutrients, on the other hand, cannot be synthesized rapidly enough or at all to meet daily needs. They must be derived from something, such as food or dietary supplements. To grow, develop, and maintain good health over the long term, your body requires six different types of essential nutrients.

1.8.1 Vitamins

Vitamins are organic chemicals found in nature that your body needs in very little amounts to function properly. Deficiencies in some nutrients mean that you must get them through food or supplements. Vitamins have an important role in digestion as well as in maintaining appropriate physiological functions.

Vitamins can be either fat- or water-soluble. When it comes to fat-soluble vitamins such as B-complex vitamins and C, there is a difference. To acquire a wide variety of vitamins, eat a diet rich in fruits, vegetables, whole grains, low-fat milk, shellfish, and eggs (Pop *et al.*, 2019).

1.8.2 Minerals

Inorganic compounds that cannot be synthesized by your body are known as minerals. Each one has a specific part in your body's regular operation as it aids in the control of biological activities. You'll need 16 minerals in your diet to sustain excellent health. Groups of people are split into two: Trace elements such as iron, zinc, iodine, selenium, copper, fluoride, chromium, molybdenum, and manganese are needed in smaller amounts by the human body compared to the other elements. Mineral-rich foods, such as fruits and vegetables, whole grains, nuts, and fortified low-fat milk, should be consumed regularly.

1.8.3 Protein

For the formation and repair of tissues in the body, protein must be present in all cells. You cannot produce all of the amino acids that make up protein in your body. As a result, protein in food is the principal supply of these essential amino acids. A complete protein has all of the body's required amino acids. Incomplete proteins, such as grains, legumes, nuts, and seeds, should be taken in a variety of ways to assure adequate intake of all necessary amino acids (Odhaib et al., 2021).

1.8.4 Fats

Monounsaturated and polyunsaturated lipids, notably omega-3 fatty acids, are important for health. According to the Harvard School of Public Health, monounsaturated and polyunsaturated fats help decrease blood cholesterol, reduce inflammation, and regulate cardiac rhythms. Omega-3 fatty acids in particular are necessary for healthy blood coagulation and brain cell membrane development. Additionally, these fatty acids may aid in the prevention of heart disease, cancer, and stroke. Foods high in healthful fats include salmon, tuna, olive oil, canola oil, flaxseed, walnuts, and almonds.

1.8.5 Carbohydrates

Although carbohydrates are not created by the body, they are broken down during digestion to provide energy for physical activity and other biological activities. Carbohydrates supply your nerves, muscles, and brain energy. According to the Harvard School of Public Health, refining complete grains into refined meals such as white bread, sweets, and white rice depletes them of minerals, fatty acids, and fiber, resulting in foods that produce larger blood sugar spikes than whole grains. Choose whole-grain slices of bread, pasta, and cereals as complex carbs, as well as nuts, beans, lentils, peas, and potatoes.

1.8.6 Water

Water makes up more than 60 percent of your body weight. Daily fluid requirements surpass what your body can produce naturally via processes such as digestion. Water is considered an essential nutrient as it is necessary for appropriate physiological function (Murdoch et al., 2000). Water carries nutrition and oxygen to cells, removes waste, maintains normal body temperature, and tones muscles and skin. Individual needs vary but consuming at least eight 8-ounce glasses of fluids every day is advisable

1.9 CONSUMPTION OF FIBER

Due to a lack of enzymes in the human stomach, dietary fiber, the structural component of plants, cannot be digested. Even though these indigestible substances, except for a small fraction that is digested by bacteria in the large intestine, pass through the gut intact, they contribute to optimum health. Insoluble fiber does not dissolve in water and offers bulk, or roughage, which aids in bowel movement and aids in the elimination of possibly carcinogenic or otherwise dangerous substances from meals.

Whole-grain slices of bread and cereals, wheat bran, and vegetables all include insoluble fiber. While soluble fiber shortens the time food travels through the stomach, which is undesirable, it also contributes to the reduction of blood cholesterol levels, which is beneficial. Gums, pectin, certain hemicelluloses, and mucilage are all soluble fibers; notable dietary sources include citrus fruits, apples, oats, barley, and legumes. Both soluble and insoluble fibers contribute to the reduction and regulation of blood glucose absorption, resulting in a slower and more balanced supply of blood glucose. Dietary fiber may protect against some gastrointestinal issues and lower the chance of developing other chronic illnesses (Multari *et al.*, 2015).

1.10 NUTRITION THAT REGULATES BODY FUNCTIONS

Without a well-balanced diet, your body cannot create all of the nutrients it requires. It is hard to go through the day without the energy that carbs and fats provide. Protein, vitamins, and water all have physiological functions in the body, and getting enough of these nutrients through your diet can help with cell function.

1.10.1 Protein

Protein is an important source of the essential amino acids that your body needs to function correctly. The body uses amino acids to produce proteins such as hemoglobin, which delivers oxygen to cells, and antibodies, which recognize and eliminate foreign particles. Protein also aids in the production of enzymes, which are proteins that perform several functions in the body. Enzymes conduct a variety of functions, including intercellular communication and energy generation. According to the United States Department of Agriculture, males should consume 56 grams of protein per day, while women should consume 46 grams.

1.11 NUTRIENTS THAT ARE SOLUBLE IN WATER

Water-soluble vitamins, such as vitamin C and the B-complex, are also required for normal cell function. Vitamin C aids in the formation of collagen, a fibrous protein that keeps cells and tissues together. The B-complex vitamins work together to break down carbs and lipids, ensuring that your cells obtain the energy they require. It's also worth noting that B-complex vitamins help your body convert protein to amino acids, which it may then employ to maintain proper cell function (Lin. *et al.*, 2010).

1.12 VITAMINS THAT MIGHT BE STORED AS FAT

The inclusion of vitamins A, E, K, and D improves your body's capacity to absorb fat-soluble vitamins. Vitamin D aids in the absorption of calcium and phosphorus, both of which are required for strong bones. Aside from kidney function, vitamin K has a direct impact on the production of cell-essential proteins. Vitamin A promotes new cell growth and development, which aids in tissue health maintenance. Vitamin E is an antioxidant that promotes tissue health in the body. Because there is no cellular damage, it avoids cell malfunction and, finally, cell death.

1.13 WATER

It is important to eat and drink sufficient water to keep your cells and tissues operating properly. Water prevents toxins from collecting and limiting cell activity by assisting your cells in removing waste materials. Water transports oxygen and nutrients to cells, allowing them to operate. It is also beneficial to avoid abnormally high or low body temperatures, which may limit enzyme action. To keep your body hydrated, men should drink at least 12 cups of water each day, while women should drink at least 9 cups per day.

1.14 IMPORTANCE OF WATER & SALT IN BODY

Water makes up the majority of the fluids that flow throughout the body. Water accounts for 45 to 75 percent of your body weight, depending on your age and muscle mass. Extracellular and intracellular fluids are present in your cells. Because salt is the most frequent ion group in extracellular fluids, it is an important electrolyte. Your kidneys control the balance of salt and water in your body (Linares et al., 2017).

1.14.1 Water is Necessary for the Body's Fluid Homeostasis to be Maintained

The appropriate balance of water and salt is critical to your health. Your kidneys perform all of the heavy labor to keep you hydrated and electrolyte-balanced. The idea is to maintain a balance between the quantity of water you ingest and the amount of water you excrete. To compensate for the loss of water in your body, your kidneys create more urine. When the volume of water is little, your kidneys are better equipped to hold it. The anti-diuretic hormone is a hormone that regulates how much water the kidneys excrete. It assists in the re-absorption of liquids, making you thirstier.

1.14.2 The Balance of Sodium and Water Osmolality is Crucial

The sodium balance must be carefully maintained to avoid any interruptions in regular cell function. Osmolality is the control of the concentration of solubilized compounds in a particular volume. Salt intake and outflow must be balanced about water intake and outflow to maintain osmolality. To prevent sodium levels from increasing during dehydration, your body must save water and eliminate salt. When you drink a lot of water, your body conserves salt to reduce sodium dilution. The salt balance in the body impacts both blood pressure and blood volume management (López *et al.*, 2019).

1.15 THE CONSEQUENCES OF SODIUM DEFICIENCY

The nervous system, muscles, and other physiological systems all require salinity to operate normally. Problems happen when your body has too much or too little sodium.

A multitude of factors can disrupt the sodium-water balance, including diuretic drugs, excessive water consumption, excessive sweating, heart failure, and renal illness. Both muscle spasms and weariness are symptoms of an imbalance.

1.16 KEEPING A LOW-SODIUM DIET

Your body's inherent checks and balances help it adjust to varied salt consumption, but lowering your sodium intake will aid in this process. Consuming too much salt can lead to high blood pressure, poor bone health, and other health problems. If your diet puts you at risk of developing high blood pressure or heart disease, limit your daily salt intake to less than 1,500 milligrams.

1.17 WATER'S VITALITY IN THE HUMAN BODY

Water is a necessary nutrient and a component of all living things. Nutrients are chemical components of food and drinks that your body need to execute metabolic and/or sustaining processes (Karioti *et al.,* 2015). To receive the nutrients your body requires, you must eat a range of foods containing these nutrients regularly.

A person who is dehydrated of any nutrient dies faster than a person who is dehydrated of water. The great bulk of human activities relies on this vital liquid.

1.18 LUBRICANT

Water's most significant purpose is as a lubricant. Saliva and the fluid that surrounds joints both contain substantial amounts of it. Water may be found in the brain, spinal cord, and eyes, for example. The aqueous layer protects these sensitive regions by acting as a buffer against the potentially fatal effects of shock and stress.

1.19 TEMPERATURE CONTROL MECHANISMS IN THE BODY

The only way to keep the body temperature stable is to drink enough water. To operate properly, the body's temperature must be regulated within a particular range.

Water helps in two ways in this process. Because water is slow to alter temperature and excellent at storing heat, the body's 60 to 75 percent water content works as a temperature regulator. This vitamin is also used by the body through sweat. Evaporation of water cools the body. It is very necessary to do so.

Protein and carbs are two of the most critical nutrients for good physiological performance. They give the vigor required for development and advancement. The cell, on the other hand, has no use for these two chemicals in the absence of water. Water facilitates the human body's digestion and use of protein and carbs (Khorram & Ramezanian, 2021).

Water is required for the body's transportation system to function properly. Every physiological action, from breathing to muscular movement to digestion and waste elimination, need the delivery of nutrients and other important components throughout the body. The human body cannot function without water.

1.20 HOW TO STAY HYDRATED

Water is necessary for your body's proper functioning, so make sure you obtain sufficient of it. Most individuals should drink eight 8-ounce glasses of water each day, however, this may vary.

You may need to drink more water if you exercise, are pregnant, or are experiencing abnormally hot weather. As a general rule, water or another beverage should be drunk throughout and between meals. Drink plenty of water before, during, and after exercise (Karthika & Sureshkumar, 2021).

Remember to drink lots of water, which is naturally present in all of your meals and beverages. Water-rich foods, such as watermelon, spinach, and celery, help you keep hydrated. You should avoid over-hydrating if you are not thirsty and your urine is pale. Drinking too much water may jeopardize your health.

1.21 FRUITS THAT BOOST ENERGY

Fruits are high in carbohydrates, vitamins, and minerals, all of which your body requires to create energy. The US Department of Agriculture suggests eating five servings of fruit every day, divided into two cups, with the quantity you consume based on your calorie needs (Karwowska et al., 2021). To reap the benefits of fiber, consume whole fruits rather than fruit juice as the majority of your daily diet. Variation is also required for your body to absorb more nutrients. If you consume the correct balance of fruits, you may feel more invigorated.

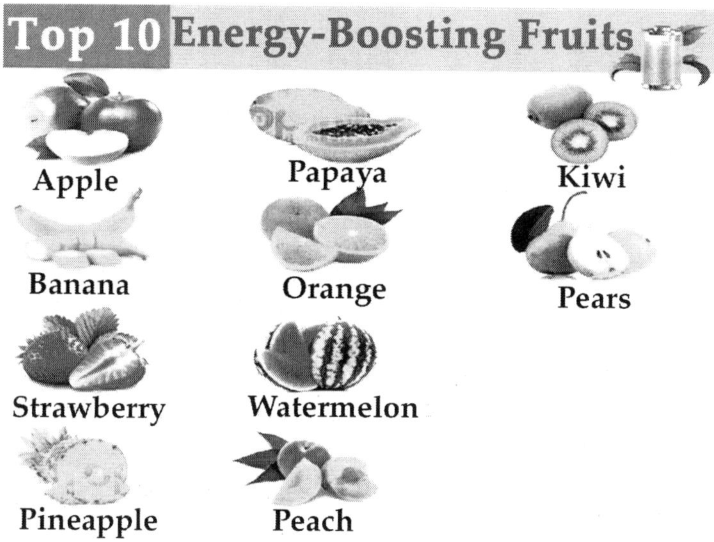

Figure 1.10: Energy-giving fruits.

Drinking water flushes toxins from the body and nourishes numerous components of the body. Dehydration, which can lead to weariness, can be avoided by drinking enough water. Including watery fruits in your diet can help you meet your daily hydration requirements. Water is included in at least 85 percent of fruits such as apples, pineapples, and apricots. The average watermelon and cantaloupe content is around 90%.

1.22 FRUITS HIGH IN CARBOHYDRATES

Carbohydrates are the body's principal source of energy. When you need a boost, your body looks to glycogen, a carbohydrate molecule generated during activity. Consuming high-carbohydrate fruits can help you maintain your energy levels and restore your glycogen reserves. Fruits' simple carbs provide a rapid source of energy for your body, as glucose is created in a short amount of time. Oranges and bananas are both heavy in carbohydrates. A cup of bananas has 34 grams of carbs while a cup of oranges contains 21 grams (Kau *et al.*, 2011).

1.23 FRUITS WITH A HIGH IRON CONTENT

Iron deficiency is characterized by a lack of energy, difficulty focusing, and an overall sense of sluggishness. Iron is required as a building ingredient for the protein hemoglobin, which delivers oxygen to cells for energy generation. Watermelons, apricots, and peaches are examples of iron-rich foods. Iron absorption is enhanced by the eating of vitamin C-rich fruits and vegetables such as apples, oranges, pineapple, and raspberries.

Here are a couple more as a follow-up.

A diet rich in fat-rich foods, antioxidants, and vitamin C will help you feel more invigorated. Avocados, for example, contain unsaturated fats, which are a fantastic source of energy, according to MayoClinic.com. Antioxidants defend against disease-causing substances that drain energy. Several fruits and vegetables are strong in antioxidants. In contrast, vitamin C increases your metabolic rate, helping you to burn more calories. Kiwi, papaya, pineapple, and watermelon, among other citrus fruits and vegetables, have high vitamin C contents. A direct calorimeter, which measures heat dissipated from a person's body, may be used to calculate energy consumption. This technology employs water-cooled clothing or insulated chambers large enough to contain a person (Kadam & Prabhasankar, 2010).

The three basic components of the human body are weight, fat, and water. Individual life events and heredity determine how much food a person consumes concerning their body composition. Water accounts for around 62 percent of a healthy lean man's body, along with 16 percent of fat and 16 percent of protein, with the remaining 6 percent of minerals and less than 1 percent of carbohydrate accounting for the remainder. The fat proportion in a healthy, slender woman is around 22 percent, whereas, in males of the same weight, the fat level is roughly 12 percent lower.

To maintain homeostasis, or dynamic balance, the body's multiple compartments, including lean body mass, body fat, and body water, continually react to changes in the internal and external environment. Catabolism and anabolism occur at varying rates in the body's tissues. Red blood cells last for 120 days, whereas connective tissue regenerates over time and digestive tract epithelial cells are replaced every three to four days (Jacob et al., 2020).

A direct inspection can identify the proportion of body fat, however, it is imprecise. DXA or direct X-ray absorptiometry can be used to quantify body fat indirectly. DXA is a time-consuming and accurate X-ray absorptiometry technology. Although less exact than anthropometry, skinfold callipers, bioelectrical resistance, and near-infrared interactants, these methods are more often used.

1.24 RECOMMENDATIONS FOR DIETARY AND NUTRIENT INTAKE

Changing times, a greater understanding of nutrition, as well as cultural and regional norms, all influence what constitutes a healthy diet. Previously, people had to rely nearly solely on food cultivated or collected in their backyards. Food can now be delivered over large distances as a result of industrialization and globalization. Because the poor cannot purchase the same foods as the wealthy, and because many nations have big immigrant groups with particular eating habits, researchers must be cautious when concluding a country's nutrition from a small sample of its population. Even in a civilized culture, some people refuse to eat certain foods for moral or religious reasons (Ibrahim *et al.*, 2015).

People in wealthier nations eat more meat and animal products in general. Agricultural countries, on the other hand, get the majority of their calories from grains like wheat flour, white rice, or corn, with just around 10% coming from animal products. Another point of distinction across civilizations is dairy products. Dairy products, for example, account for around 2% of China's energy use. Dairy products, on the other hand, account for more than 10% of Pakistan's energy use. The Mediterranean diet, on the other hand, has the fewest saturated fats of any Western diet. Despite limited medical treatment and low living standards, Europeans in rural areas surrounding the Mediterranean Sea had a higher life expectancy in the 1950s than those in other parts of Europe. In the traditional Mediterranean diet, olive oil is the primary source of monounsaturated fats, which are abundant in the diet while being low in animal products. Tomatoes and leafy green vegetables include a variety of antioxidants that have been linked to increased health in the region.

Genetics tend to have the greatest effect on a person's life expectancy, regardless of how healthy they are. Despite this, healthy lifestyle choices including limiting alcohol use, stopping smoking, and engaging in regular physical activity may help to minimize early mortality and improve long-term health. Our energy requirements change as we age, so it's critical to consume a diet that's excellent for adults in general.

Due to a multitude of circumstances, including tooth loss, loss of taste and odor, and social isolation, the elderly are more prone to suffer from poor nutrition. Elderly persons are more prone to experience digestive problems such as constipation and insufficient vitamin B12 absorption. You may become dehydrated if you do not drink enough water. Nutritional deficiencies can hasten the aging of the immune system. The use of prescription and over-the-counter medications can worsen geriatric nutritional deficiencies. A lack of physical activity, as well as muscle loss, has been linked to type 2 diabetes, hypertension, cardiovascular disease, and other diseases. Individuals over the age of 65 may require additional vitamin D to maintain bone density, especially if they do not consume enough fatty fish or vitamin D-rich meals. While taking adequate calcium and engaging in weight-bearing workouts are vital, they cannot prevent bone density loss, which raises the risk of fractures in both men and women as they age. You may become dehydrated if you do not drink enough water. Nutritional deficiencies can hasten the aging of the immune system. The use of prescription and over-the-counter medications can worsen geriatric nutritional deficiencies. A lack of physical activity, as well as muscle loss, has been linked to type 2 diabetes, hypertension, cardiovascular disease, and other diseases. Individuals over the age of 65 may require additional vitamin D to maintain bone density, especially if they do not consume enough fatty fish or vitamin D-rich meals (Hou & Xu, 2022).

The benefits of calcium and weight-bearing exercise cannot be emphasized; yet, these measures will not prevent bone density loss as people age, putting them in danger of osteoporosis-related bone fractures that can leave them bedridden or even dead. A variety of bone-preserving medications have been demonstrated to reduce bone loss. Healthy aging may help people prevent falls, enhance their general well-being, and reduce the severity of chronic conditions like osteoporosis, which can lead to bed rest or even death if left untreated. There are a variety of drugs that have been demonstrated in recent research to decrease bone loss. Staying physically healthy as we age may help us preserve our strength and balance, as well as our general health and well-being.

Age-related macular degeneration, the most prevalent cause of blindness in those over 65, can be delayed by taking vitamins C, E, beta-carotene, and zinc. Researchers are studying lutein to understand more about how these carotenoids might help maintain our eyesight sharper as we age. According to the study, people with osteoarthritis may benefit from consuming glucosamine, a naturally occurring chemical that aids in the development of cartilage. Physical activity, weight loss, and strength training can all help to alleviate arthritis discomfort.

It is critical to maintain a nutritious diet, get enough sleep, avoid smoking, exercise, and keep your mind busy if you want to live a long life in your elderly years (Haque et al., 2020). The so-called "free-radical theory of aging," which claims that highly reactive substances damage cellular components and that antioxidant intake can repair this damage and thus slow aging, has sparked considerable interest and is a promising area of research, but it has yet to be scientifically established. Antioxidant treatment, on the other hand, has not considerably increased the life duration of numerous mammalian species. Nonhuman primates are being examined to determine if undernutrition, rather than hunger, slow the aging process and increases life spans. Extreme energy restriction appears to have little effect on life expectancy beyond the existing range of 115–120 years.

1.25 SUGGESTIONS FOR VITAMIN AND MINERAL SUPPLEMENTATION IN THE DIET

Governments typically seek dietary advice from scientific groups within their boundaries. The World Health Organization and other United Nations entities have also published information on nutrients and dietary components. The RDAs (Recommended Dietary Allowances) were created by the National Academy of Sciences in the United States in 1941 and were reviewed regularly until 1989, creating dietary guidelines to measure population nutritional intakes and manage food supply. The RDAs reflected the best scientific judgment available at the time for determining the amount of each nutrient required to fulfill the dietary needs of the vast majority of healthy people.

CHAPTER 2

TRENDS IN HUMAN NUTRITION

CONTENTS

2.1 SUSTAINABLE AND ENVIRONMENTAL FRIENDLY NUTRITION

A sustainable diet is defined as one that is generally healthy and has minimal effects on the food supply and the environment in general. The adoption of a sustainable diet is useful in maintaining an individual's health while ensuring that the planet has enough resources needed to feed future generations of human beings. The main aim of adopting sustainable and environment-friendly nutrition is to ensure the effects on human health and the environment are positive. Current research shows that food production is among the largest causes of global environmental changes. Studies show that the adoption of vegan and vegetarian diets is useful in reducing land use and the amount of greenhouse gas emissions (Halloran et al., 2015). Such kinds of diets are known to use little amounts of water. The universally healthy reference diet is made up of legumes, nuts, whole grains, fruits, and vegetables. The adoption of a sustainable diet involves the reduction of the consumption of processed foods, red meat, added sugars, and refined grain.

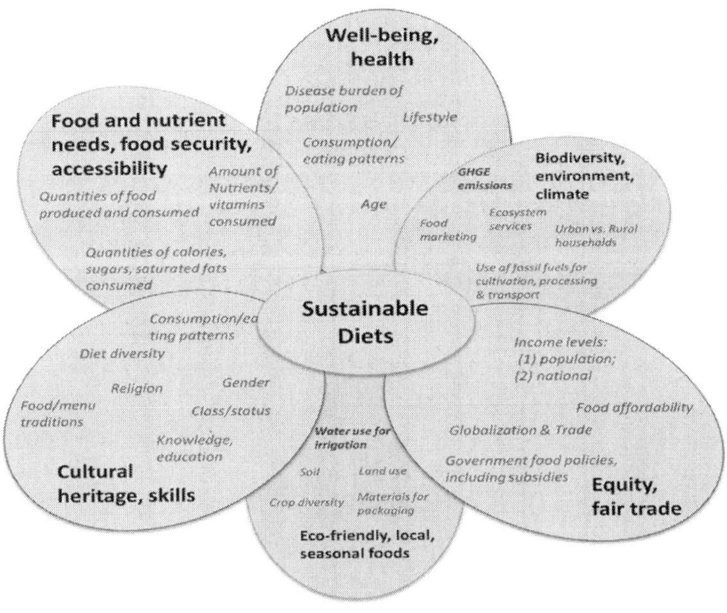

Figure 2.1: A sustainable diet will be able to support large numbers of human populations.

(Source: Miller KB, Eckberg JO , 2021)

A truly sustainable diet places much emphasis on the health of the environment. Such diets consider the general effects on the environment and the individual and the food chain in general. Some of the factors taken into consideration when formulating such a diet include general health, ecosystem protection, biodiversity, relative cost, and nutritional availability. Taking the factors into consideration will be useful in ensuring the provision of food and resources for a growing population. Sustainable and environmentally friendly nutrition is mostly found in vegetarian and plant-based diets. When compared to diets containing meat, they are found to be more sustainable. Studies show that plant-based food cause few adverse effects on the environment. Among the topics of conversation when developing a sustainable diet is the incorporation of animal products such as eggs, dairy, and meat. There are a few significant impacts to be taken into consideration with animal products. They include greenhouse emissions, water use, and land use.

There is still a place for animal food in a sustainable diet. The major challenge is to agree on how much animal food a person can eat while maintaining sustainability. Under the adoption of sustainable diets, it was noted that consumers have a preference for food products with little or no packaging more so those from local and social businesses. Here is an increased preference for regularly and seasonally grown vegetables and fruits. Some opt to grow their diets on their own (Hathwar *et al.,* 2012).

2.2 VEGAN AND PLANT-BASED NUTRITION

Vegan and plant-based diets have been adopted to eliminate all animal products. Plant-based diets however have been made with the aim of not necessarily eliminating animals but placing much emphasis on eating mostly plants such as whole grains, seeds, vegetables, and fruits. While adopting a vegan diet, the individual eliminates all animal products such as honey, eggs, fish, poultry, meat, and dairy. There are various reasons why people choose to follow a vegan diet. They include health reasons and environmental or ethical reasons. Adoption of a vegan diet has several health benefits. However, there are some pitfalls to avoid. Just because the diet is entirely plant-based it does not necessarily is healthy. A person may be vegan and still eat vegan junk foods, potato chips, and vegan cookies. Some of these foods may be high in calories but very low in nutrients. For this reason, it is very advisable to eat whole foods.

A plant-based diet however leaves the individual free to decide whether or not they would want to consume animal products. A major focus is placed on eating foods that are plant sources. Plant-based diets usually place much emphasis on the consumption of whole food. This means that food has been subjected to minimal processing and is very close to its natural state (Ferreira & Nunes, 2019). Some examples of plant-based foods include nuts, seeds, plant-based oils such as avocado, olive, and canola, whole grains such as barley, farro, and oatmeal, and fruits and vegetables. With vegetable and plant-based diets, there is a need for one to develop a meal plan. The main component of a meal plan requires that it is made up of 50% vegetables. Although fruits are good, much emphasis is placed on the consumption of vegetables as they have little amounts of sugar.

Three main things that guide the plate-building process include having 50% vegetables, 25% lean protein, and 25% whole grains. If an individual wants to eat meat occasionally, they should stick to eating lean poultry, fish, and meat. Such diets may allow the adoption of healthy fats such as avocado when roasting vegetables. By adding healthy fat, the diet is very nutritious. Nutrition experts have observed vegan and plant-based nutrition. They anticipate that it will move to the mass markets with so much demand being placed on vegan convenience products more so those that have been packed in environmentally sustainable packaging. It is also expected that vegan and plant-based diets will expand to the field of sports and nutrition and eventually into clinical nutrition. There has been a noticeable increase in the demand for high-quality vegan supplements (Francesconi, 2007).

2.3 PERSONALIZED NUTRITION AND BIOHACKING

Personalization nutrition is a philosophy that transforms attitudes to drinks and foods. Some of the information said to be very important is the sensitivities and the biological effect. They may even out-weigh questions of ethics, convenience, and taste. There is a current trend where people see food as medicine and also as a substance causing food and beverage companies to administer to their new-found needs. Personalization in nutrition started in medicine with treatments and drugs adapted to suit the person's predicted response or risk of disease based on genetic makeup. This to the long-term trend in nutrition more so with the biohacker to the fore. In the future, there may be hyper-personalized diets made up of functional food recommendations formed based on scientific testing.

It has been noted that a large number of people are leaning towards the use of personalized nutrition. This has been linked to the increase in allergies, intolerance, and the great desire to optimize body performance. This has led to consumers opting to consult their nutritionist. Based on the needs of the body and the individual's preference, the nutritionist will develop a suitable diet that will ensure the individual is not missing out on any kind of nutrients even though some foods have been eliminated from their diet (Fabani et al., 2013). Some can formulate their personalized diets by utilizing the information they get from wearable devices and apps. Both the apps and devices are fitted with information on various food choices. Biohacking is also a part of nutrition. It is said to be beyond food intake.

Among the desire of people is to be the best version of themselves. Biohacking goes further as it facilitates the adoption of a systems-thinking approach to their biology. It involves taking into consideration everything that is placed into the body. This ranges from foods and drinks to ideas and movement. They affect the outcome whether it is a disease, athletics, weight, performance in business and energy. Biohacking is useful in transforming the inner workings which leaves the body more energized, more productive and the individual feels like they are the best version of themselves. This trend can be taken to the extreme by the biohackers themselves availing themselves of CRISPR, the cheap and relatively easy technique for making precise changes to DNA.

Nutritionists have noticed an increased range of tailored nutrition concepts that range from listening to the body's nutrition concepts and using technology such as gut microbe analysis or DNA tests. There are several benefits of the concept of personalized eating including making eating more fun and enjoyable and also improving the health and well-being of the individual.

2.4 NUTRITION CONFUSION

With so much information on nutrition available on the internet, it leaves people confused as they may not know the most appropriate diet that suits them. There are different diets, plans, and recipes o stick to. There are different topics under nutrition confusion which includes carbon confusion. The choice of the type of carbohydrates to incorporate into a diet is known to generate great controversy. The newest thing is the adoption of low-carb diets (Dixon & Sumner, 2003). The choice of the type of carbohydrates to incorporate into the die has been controlled by studies on the difference between high-carbohydrate diets and low-carbohydrate diets. It has proven to contribute to the success and sustainability of the diet. It was noted that problems related to health are noted when they heavily rely on refined carbohydrate foods.

As nutrient confusion may be a major challenge to the lives of consumers, they are advised to take the entire process personally. This is because the type of diet they would want to adopt should be compatible with their body. This is useful in ensuring that the individual gets the results they require.

There are several cases where people adopt new information about food that they stop consuming foods that they consumed initially. Those alterations may not result in the changes they wanted.

There was a time when people heard that eating gluten would make people sick causing people to avoid wheat-based foods. People should not be jumping on every new trend. Before the nutrition plan is adopted, the individual should conduct suitable research. This may involve them consulting their dietician or nutritionist who will conduct tests on their body to establish the appropriate kind of diet to take up.

2.5 PREVENTION THROUGH NUTRITION EDUCATION

In the nutrition world, there has been an increased demand for dietetic treatment more so in clinics where the demand has not been met as a result of financial resources. It was also noted that consumers have become increasingly aware that investing in nutrition education among children is an important tool used in fostering healthy habits at a young age. Experts also observed that health and nutrition education in companies has shifted from solely being focused on physical activity to a very holistic approach.

Under this, the most important topics are nutrition and mindfulness. Nutritionists place much emphasis on the need for successful nutrition communication for a healthy diet to be easy to understand for everyone (Da Silva et al., 2016).

There is a great need for recommendations and recipes being close to everyday life. They should also be very easy to implement. It was noted that most parents want learning institutions to be a place for nutrition education by promoting healthy meals for their children.

2.6 ALTERNATIVE PROTEINS

It was noted that large numbers of people are opting to replace meat as a source of protein in their diet. This has led to the adoption of alternative sources of protein which are mostly plant-based. They, therefore, include food products made from plants such as nuts, legumes, and grains. Some alternative proteins are derived from cultured meat, insects, algae, and fungus. Several claims have been put forward by companies involved in the production of alternative proteins. Depending on the type of product, the alternative protein can simulate the texture and taste of conventional meat (Dayan et al., 2009). The claim is that since the benefits of alternative proteins combine with the environment and human beings, they encourage new technologies and businesses which contribute to the economic pillar of sustainable development. The challenge is ha most of these claims are usually unsubstantiated and may lack supporting evidence. The adoption of plant-based proteins has been quite popular as it is viewed to be a more healthy alternative. Most companies use that as a strategy to build their sales. Much emphasis has been placed on the need for these products to be produced with minimal processes.

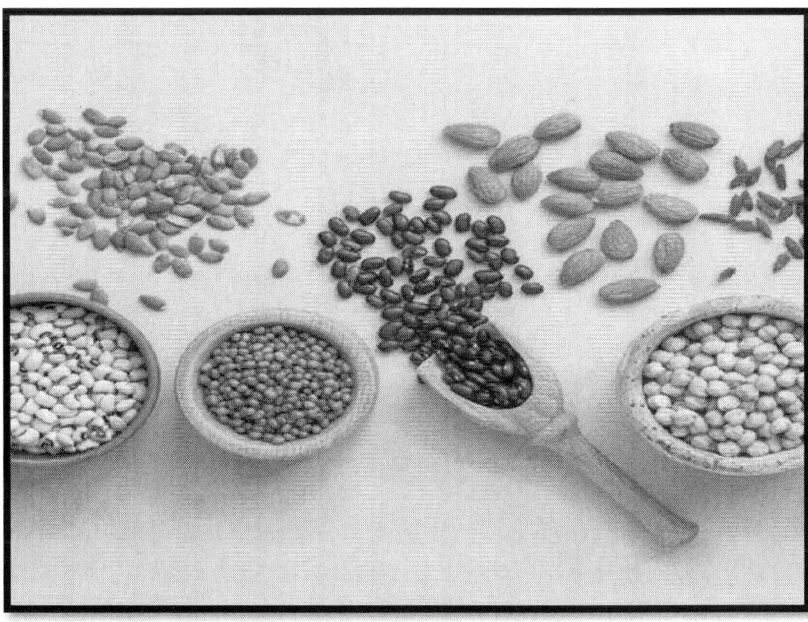

Figure 2.2: Plant-based proteins are a good protein alternative.

2.7 MINDFUL EATING AND HEALTH AT EVERY SIZE

There was a decade that was entirely characterized by the yo-yo effect, dieting, and counting calories. Currently, the food trend involves fewer food bans and more fun and relaxed approaches to the type of nutrition adopted. In this trend, mindful eating and health at every stage are very important. Some companies and nutritionists help people of all sizes find compassionate ways of ensuring that they take care of themselves. A good example is HAES which led to the development of fat acceptance and body positivity movement. There are various effects on health at every step and there are certain interventions that have to be made on health-related outcomes for people with obesity and overweight. The concept of mindful eating has been used to actively describe one paying attention to food eaten, moment by moment without judgment. Mindful eating and health at every step place much focus on the individual itself and his/her intuition. This leads to a sustainable and positive mindset. Some individuals believe having breakfast that might be the most important meal of the day while other people believe breakfast is not important. This can lead to the conclusion of less compulsion and more pleasure (Caporgno & Mathys, 2018). There is significant evidence to show that weight loss interventions through behavioral modification, exercise, and dietary restriction have mostly failed. Popularity is mostly with regards to health at every size moment. Many nutritionists have made it their mission to promote the weight-neutral approach for more health and well-being in a given area.

2.8 NUTRIENTS ON THE GO AND MEAL REPLACEMENT

There have been notable changes in traditional food habits more so in modern families. This mostly includes both parents working which leads to full-time care for children in kindergarten and school. Previously, the most important meal in families was lunch. There were times when it was breakfast and now its dinner. Therefore, there is an increased search for meal replacement and the nutrient on the go may support them during long working hours. They may also be able to follow a healthy diet that is rich in nutrients. The nutrient on the go is made up of solutions that provide supplements or food based on natural ingredients useful in enhancing the body's performance. There are private dietetic consultations where clients are observed to request nutritious meal replacements that they can integrate into their busy lives.

2.9 KETOGENIC NUTRITION

A broad range of consumers has been made to make use of ketogenic diets. It was noted that for population groups such as athletes, there is a growing trend where they minimize the number of supplements ingested while implementing specific diets in their place. An example of such a diet is the ketogenic diet. This kind of diet is a high-fat, low-carbohydrate but normal protein diet which forces the body to burn at a faster rate compared to carbohydrates in energy generation (Cassani et al., 2020). The ketogenic diet is a classic therapeutic diet that was developed for the treatment of pediatric epilepsy in the 1920s. Some of the benefits of the diet include it being used in treating patients suffering from acne, Alzheimer and multiple sclerosis. The ketogenic diet has been well established in sports nutrition and bodybuilding. What has been observed is amateur sportsmen who are requesting more information about it facilitating the ketogenic diet in training plans.

2.10 SUGAR-FREE NUTRITION

In the current day and age, many parents have become more informed on the adverse effect of products with high amounts of sugar. There is a great desire for healthy eating habits which led to the anti-sugar movement. The movement has continued for longer durations and still needs to. This is often at times accompanied by evidence-based campaigns educating children and parents about sweeteners, sugar substitutes, and sugar. This kind of information is very useful for children as they are more prone to consume much sugar in their diets through drinks or snacks. Nutritionists noted that as they interacted with families, the families demonstrated the desire to provide healthy meals to their kids. This places much need for parents to get needed support to understand the amount of sugar in different products and their effects.

2.11 BOTANICAL BOOM

The term botanical is a term used to refer to plant-derived extracts greatly used medicinally for several years. Among the latest trends is that there is a great desire for natural plant-based products while increasing the overall health and emotional well-being have contributed to the popularity of botanicals in food, beverage, and supplements worldwide. It is important to ensure that the quality and safety of botanicals are well maintained. This is to deal with safety concerns (Bulaj et al., 2016). There are regulatory bodies such as the EFSA that seek to guide science-based safety assessment as well as a compendium of botanicals all of which have reported safety concerns. For this reason, the method of extraction is a very important consideration for the safety and quality of the botanical and also the taste of the final product. Currently, science is still trying to catch up to the perceptions of consumers for many botanical all of which makes claims challenging.

CHAPTER 3

SOURCES OF FOOD

CONTENTS

3.1 INTRODUCTION

Food is a necessity for survival. Humans have always relied on natural sources for nourishment. Rapid population expansion, especially in the last few years, has necessitated an increase in food supply to keep up with demand. However, the focus has been on providing staple meals rather than a comprehensive diet that includes a variety of foods that offer the many ingredients that the body needs for healthy functioning. Foods, whether from nonindigenous or indigenous sources, undergo a series of phases to become available for consumption, which is governed by culture, technology, and the economic system (Bis-Souza et al., 2019). Some of these elements have an impact on the long-term viability of food supplies. Nutrients and some non-nutrient found in meals are required for development and physiological functioning, according to advances in nutritional and food sciences. Because certain meals contain more (types and quantities of) nutrients and non-nutrient than others, eating a variety of foods is necessary to meet the body's demands.

Because various elements coexist in meals, their interactions must be understood, and the balancing of constituents is required for optimal health benefits. Furthermore, many food sources must be discovered, made available, and eaten to maintain a healthy lifestyle. The different roles of nutritional and non-nutrient substances in foods are required for growth and well-being in health. As a result, both the amount and quality of food sources must be examined, and both will be explored in the context of long-term food sources (Ambuja & Rajakumar, 2018).

In human history, natural foods have supplied the wherewithal to sustain life. Indigenous people rely heavily on indigenous foods found in their environment, which they get by gathering and hunting. On land, the forest is the primary food supply, with foods from streams supplementing it. People who live along the coast have access to the water or ocean, which is another big natural source of food. The survival of plants or animals in the soil and climatic conditions of the area determines the food variety and breeds chosen. Amaranths, corn (maize), squashes (*Cucurbita* spp.), and beans (*Phaseolus* spp.), were discovered as weeds in areas cultivated with cassava and sweet potato.

In general, crops that began as weeds have gone through three phases before becoming human food sources. They were first removed, sliced, or dug into the earth, but as weeds grew, some were able to endure and survive. Farmers began planting after weeds had been with them long enough for them to understand their value. In traditional agricultural communities, getting food and gathering wood for the fire were the most important occupations. For both food and non-food producers, agricultural development made life simpler and far less time-consuming to acquire food supply.

The very first animals kept in animal husbandry were most likely chickens, ducks, pigs, sheep, rabbits, goats, and cattle. They were a source of both food and non-food resources. Food is mostly provided by poultry and small animals, while draft animals supply both food and power. When the supply power, however, consumes around 20% of the farm's entire agricultural yield. The use of such animal power to pull a plow and, subsequently, the advent of tractors, were agricultural productivity breakthroughs. Keeping herds of animals for food and other purposes ensured the food supply was secure.

Trading for food is also popular in traditional civilization, with food for food and food for nonfood things being the most common methods. Foods can be exchanged through a monetary exchange in a cash economic model or less conventional settings. Foods may be transferred away from their native locations and thus become non-indigenous to the new locations, thanks to technological advancements and communication tools (Bacon & Hobson, 2014). These foods might be just as significant as native cuisine. Immigrants transfer new cuisines and dietary practices, as well as a food culture, from one society to another, or mix it with the existing culture. Furthermore, indigenous people may accept the new cultures brought in by outsiders and make them their own. Globalization and economic liberalization have resulted in fast mobility of food (animal and plant sources) from location to location. In rare circumstances, such as limited production or recurring natural disasters, the same foodstuff as the indigenous item may be brought in from elsewhere.

3.2 FOOD SOURCES

3.2.1 Indigenous Food Sources

Wild vegetation and animals were the staple diet before official crop development. Plants and animals native to the area were harvested locally or hunted in neighboring woods and streams. Food plants that grow spontaneously in the wilderness or near the farmhouse are known as wild food plants. Sorghum, cassava, finger millet, and a variety of fruits and vegetables, for example, are natural food sources in Africa.

Plants or animals ingested by indigenous peoples in the region might be considered traditional or indigenous food sources. Several plants traditionally consumed in Africa have high nutritional value. Young stems or leaves, flowers, and fruits are edible components that can be eaten raw, cooked as side dishes, or garnished. It's possible that they are only available during certain seasons, or that various portions are used in various seasons. These plants might come from a farm or a backyard garden, as well as natural sources (Ballester-Sánchez *et al.,* 2019). According to in-depth research conducted in a rural community in northeastern Thailand, 126 food items were collected from the forest and fields at various periods throughout the year. These included insects, frogs, ground lizards, and freshwater algae, as well as foods from unusual sources including insects, amphibians, and ground lizards.

Hunger is steadily rising again after decades of reduction. One out of every five persons in Africa is malnourished. The 2030 Agenda for Sustainable Development emphasizes the battle for food and nutrition security. Donors, governments, and corporations are focusing their efforts on crop types, agricultural inputs, and technology advancements. A collection of research initiatives sponsored by the Food & Business Research Program took a different approach: promoting local and indigenous foods and crops by using traditional knowledge and technology, as well as local farmers' and communities' 'local food plates.

Numerous indigenous foods and manufacturing methods may help people get more micronutrients in their diets. Green leafy plants including *Vigna unguiculata, Hibiscus sabdariffa, Amaranthus* spp., *Solanum americanum, Solanum scabrum, Basella* spp., *Bidens pilosa, Corchorus* spp., *Gynandropsis* spp., and *Celosia* spp., thrive wild in humid tropical areas. They are traditionally eaten as leafy greens. Knowing that these leaves are rich sources of protein, phosphate, iron, vitamins A and C, and potentially vitamin B and that they are routinely consumed in regular meals, makes their usage an appealing method to enhance diets. Several traditional plants have been utilized for medical purposes in addition to their usage as meals. Efforts are being conducted across the world to discover and quantify the active components in indigenous foods that may have biologically beneficial health qualities (Ananda et al., 2017).

Encouraging indigenous foods has two significant social benefits: they are wholesome and nutritious meals that are cheap to the poor, and they may empower producers and manufacturers, who are frequently women.

Because indigenous foods are associated with traditional knowledge, their promotion may increase respect for people's cultural identities. The absence of scientific understanding about the nutritional content of many indigenous foods, as well as appropriate processing and preservation methods, is a major impediment to realizing these societal advantages. The Food & Business research programs made significant contributions in this area.

The nutritional content (micro and macronutrients, acids, proteins, vitamins, and minerals) of over 300 plant foods, vegetables, grains, seeds, and animal resources (like insects, snails, and fish) were examined and reported in Zambia, Benin, and Kenya. Based on the findings, a Zambian hospital experimented with treating critically malnourished newborns using mabisi, a local fermented milk product. New preservation techniques discovered in Kenya improved not just the shelf life but also the nutritional content of local vegetables.

Indigenous and local food promotions have the potential to enhance the livelihood of small-scale entrepreneurs and farmers who cultivate, prepare, and market these foods. Growing and preparing indigenous foods provided women in Benin and Kenya with a greater and more consistent income (Ananda *et al.,* 2017). Furthermore, there are several options for the partnership for better value chain governance, such as with farmer cooperatives, women's organizations, youth organizations, local seed banks, or consumer organizations.

There are, however, significant obstacles that the initiatives addressed. A lack of certified and dependable production and processing methods is a hindrance for small farmers who want to expand their products beyond the family and informal market (required for quality consistency). The findings of the study helped to improve parboiled rice processing procedures in Benin and vegetable drying techniques in Kenya. Another stumbling block is that most indigenous foods and crops are not certified. Working collaboratively with government authorities, two initiatives achieved significant milestones: in Benin, a newly formulated infant formula was approved and is now available for purchase in shops; in Uganda, indigenous vegetable seedlings were given enhanced legal status (Yousuf et al., 2021).

Indigenous foods can improve ecological sustainability by making contributions to plant biodiversity, strengthening resilience to climate change (for example, due to genetic diversity within farmer varieties of indigenous plants), and requiring fewer natural resources than commercial and densely farmed crops. Indigenous vegetables, which may be harvested more times per year than many other crops, also help farmers who are more likely to have failed harvests as a result of climate change.

Several initiatives provided valuable insights into the use of natural fertilizers and pest management methods, water conservation approaches, and the conservation of local forest resources, even though these environmental advantages were not the major study aims. More study on the potential environmental advantages of indigenous foods is needed, especially when local farmers' knowledge of how to raise and preserve these crops is dwindling.

Freshwater fish, frogs, crabs, and shrimp, are essential animal protein sources in addition to vegetables. The annual rainfall is when food is most plentiful. Some crops and animals can also be preserved for food. Plants are accessible from domestic activities and a few from the forest during the chilly, dry season, which corresponds with rice harvest time. Plants are mostly accessible from home gardening during the hot, dry season (Walker et al., 2015). Other potential sources are nearby rivers or local marketplaces. Seasonality influences, not just the food products, but also the manner of food acquisition in northeastern Benin. When the household's stock of staples was limited, gifts and purchased meals played a big role.

Despite the existing understanding of the nutritional content and quality of meals that may be constructed to satisfy the nutritional demands of indigenous peoples, there is a definite need to promote the use of indigenous sources. Food production should transition from focusing on commercially valuable commodities to increasing the utilization of indigenous food sources. As a result, the effort will be focused on discovering healthy indigenous food sources, as well as improving the quality and quantity of indigenous food sources. Medicinal characteristics should also be investigated to better understand their health advantages.

3.2.2 Food from Natural Waters

Capture fisheries have a long history in the SW Indian Ocean, where they are vital to coastal people's food security and culture. Mariculture, on the other hand, is a relatively young industry with few profitable commercial operations, and many projects remain primitive and subsistence-level. In recent decades, population pressure along the southwest Indian Ocean coast, along with declining nearshore fish supplies, has emerged as a possible danger to food security (Vanbergen & Initiative, 2013). Regional nations, like many other poor countries across the world, have limited economic growth options and rely mainly on basic natural resources. Because individuals lack alternative skills or possibilities to earn a livelihood, fishing is often the last choice as a result of a low Human Development Index (UNDP 2013).

Half of the world's coastal resources are in moderate to high danger of deterioration, according to the World Resources Institute (WRI). Industrial, urban, and agricultural pollutants, landfill, river damming and diversion, mangrove clearing, sedimentation, mining, and oil drilling and recovery are all quickly degrading coastal fish habitats. Marine fish output can only be increased if fish populations are regenerated and the marine food chain's equilibrium is restored. Environmental deterioration also affects inland waters, resulting in reduced catches and smaller fish. Aggressive fishing tactics and serious deterioration of marine and coastal habitats have overexploited the natural fish species.

Bottom trawls, dredges, and explosives, as well as anchoring of ships, are all fishing activities that have negative effects on aquatic environments. Large quantities of by-catch (unintended catch, nontargeted fish, or undersized fish) of juveniles of commercial species can cause significant damage since it affects the future amount of adult fish. It's critical to devise a plan for reducing bycatch and discard losses. In heavily populated coastal and fertile offshore areas, overfishing is particularly serious (Turner & Thompson, 2013).

The extent of global cooperation and governments' willingness to manage their fishing fleets are critical to the success of control measures. Since the early 1970s, the United Nations has been working to reach an agreement on how member nations should share ocean resources fairly. Despite the failure of the endeavor, numerous nations with significant coastline interests proclaimed unilateral 200-mile economic zones. Increased income and catch quantities should be the outcome of better management. However, even with competent management, these strategies will only avoid a long-term fall in capture fisheries productivity rather than delivering a substantial gain. In underdeveloped nations, fish is a key protein source and a good source of micronutrients, although consumption is substantially lower than in developed countries.

Wherever feasible, solutions to the most pressing challenges are proposed, with the goal that governments would be able to apply these suggestions to ensure long-term food security from ocean biodiversity. Given the wide variety of fisheries in the SW Indian Ocean region, as well as the high complexity of species, user groups, scientific evaluation, and environmental sustainability, this will not be a simple feat. When authorities fail to appropriately manage the number of fishers, methods utilized, and harvest volumes, overfishing of marine resources becomes a severe problem. Limiting harvests is impossible without considerable social, economic, and political disruption, as well as the availability of alternative livelihood options, given the heavy reliance of coastal people on fisheries for food security and economic activity. As a result, even in the face of substantial evidence of overfishing, there is an insufficient political will to achieve change, which is exacerbated by a lack of other livelihood alternatives (Tang *et al.,* 2020).

Extending coastal fishing into deeper seas is commonly mentioned as a way to boost sea harvests. Deep-sea bottom fish, on the other hand, are notoriously difficult to exploit sustainably under current economic conditions and governance systems, owing to their sluggish growth and poor productivity. Before investing in new fishing fleets or infrastructure, it is critical to perform assessments of the structure and biomass of possible deep-water resources. The lack of national research infrastructure in most regional nations to assess deep-water fishing resources remains a barrier to their growth; however, this might be remedied by leasing survey boats.

Only a small percentage of species and fisheries have successful management strategies. Sector management plans have been produced and even gazetted in numerous nations, but they have yet to be completely executed after several years. This might be due to a lack of institutional capability and political will, as well as apprehension about how to turn a plan into active management procedures in some circumstances.

Almost the majority of the nations bordering the SW Indian Ocean lack the data and knowledge necessary to accurately define their fisheries and the human stresses on stocks. Basic data on fished species is lacking, and additional information is needed to characterize distribution patterns, biological traits and reference points, stock conditions, and fishing impacts (Stintzing & Carle, 2004). Recent regional efforts have made significant progress in consolidating existing fisheries data and supporting research on major exploited species. These studies should be continued, and the data they provide should be included in fisheries management plans.

The relationship between research and management is frequently broken, resulting in studies that are not prioritized, such as those to predict stock status or propose answers to recent or long-standing management challenges. Studies have been conducted in certain circumstances, but their findings have not been adequately conveyed or applied. Within a governance structure, the science/management interface may be enhanced, for example, by frequent meetings between executives and scientists to discuss management needs and assist lead research activities. A vital link might be regional and national processes for reviewing the integration of scientific discoveries into management.

A noteworthy beneficial development in the SW Indian Ocean is the increased knowledge and application of an ecosystem strategy to fisheries management (EAF). The use of ecological indicators to assess and compare the state of exploited marine ecosystems (such as the Indi-seas project) is also promising. Both systems are relatively new to the region and are backed by governments; nevertheless, by making them appealing among coastal communities, their implementation may be hastened and established over a larger base. To foster acceptance and support at the community level, the positive effects of EAF management must be proved to stakeholders, particularly in the artisanal fishing industry.

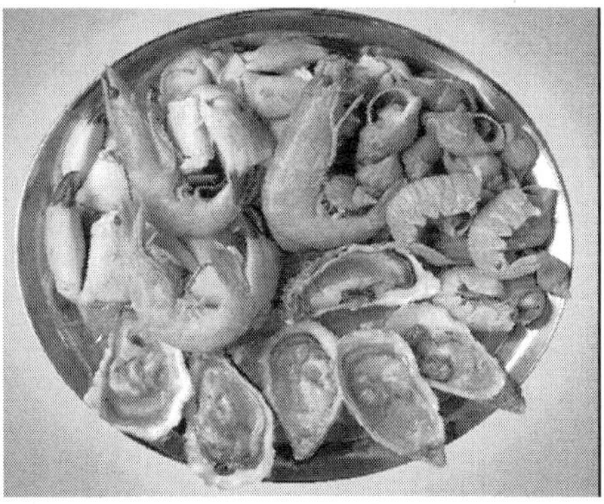

Figure 3.1: Wild seafood is often harvested by fishing or hunting.

Transboundary fish populations in the SW Indian Ocean include highly migratory billfish and tunas that travel great distances over high seas and EEZ areas, as well as more stationary species like benthic crustaceans that are found across geopolitical borders. The Indian Ocean Tuna Commission, of which many SW Indian Ocean nations are members, manages international fisheries for big pelagic species in the Indian Ocean. Through alongshore migration or larval dispersal in ocean currents, benthic populations (such as prawns) may be shared across geopolitical boundaries. As a result, one country's harvesting efforts may have an impact on another's chances (Shipp & Abdel-Aal, 2010).

Governments promote mariculture as a viable option for generating fish protein and revenue. It's a complicated developing issue that encompasses everything from land and sea-use planning to identifying the correct species and cultural technologies, as well as promoting responsible practices. To support and encourage prospective farmers, better governance systems are required. With the exception of seaweed farming in Zanzibar, project implementation and donor-driven mariculture programs have largely been short-lived and have had little acceptance. While the barriers to sustainability may vary (e.g., a lack of skills, equipment, infrastructure, marketing, etc.), the distance of much of the region from big metropolitan centers and overseas markets appears to be a common issue. Local marketing remains the major driver for mariculture – although it is less appealing than capture fishing – due to a lack of access to markets for cultivated products and effective distribution networks.

Sea cucumber farms in southwest Madagascar, where the partnership between farmers (raising), NGOs (technology), and business (marketing) has proven effective over multiple years, demonstrate the need for a more integrated approach to mariculture. Donor and/or private sector funding would be required in such a system over a long period, with a gradual provision of training. Mariculture has the potential to empower women in both cultural and commercial aspects. Seaweed farming in Zanzibar is a good example of this, and it's expected to spread across the area as more mariculture initiatives are developed. Mariculture, which starts from a low foundation and is typically backed by local communities, investors, NGOs, and governments, has unquestionably great development potential in the area over the next decade. To allow for the sector's expansion, the sector's growth constraints (such as a lack of skills, technology, and infrastructure; accessibility to markets; burdensome governance structures; and planning) must be recognized and solved.

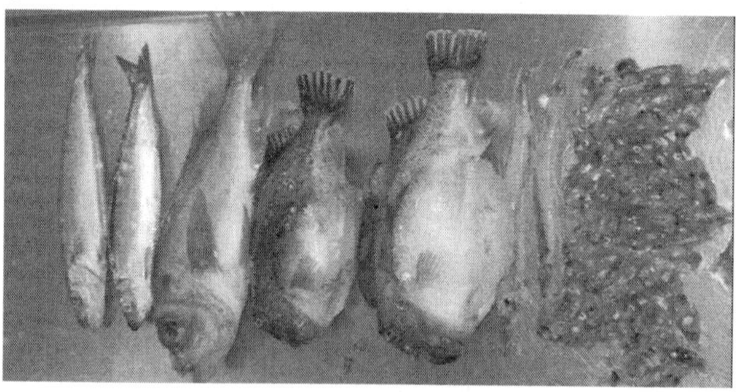

Figure 3.2: The ocean, especially via the spread of marine aquaculture.

Ironically, the tremendous biodiversity of this tropical region, as well as the range of ways utilized to utilize the marine and coastal environment for food and economic activity, is the source of several governance issues. In most cases, only a few governance resources are available to solve these complicated concerns. Nonetheless, over the last decade, significant progress has been made: governance systems have been established; capacity building is progressing; governments have signed international treaties; a shift toward EAF rather than single-species management; co-management through the development of BMUs; implications of research and management; and the recognition that mariculture will be critical to food security, social and economic systems shortly (Sharma *et al*., 2021). Governments in the SW Indian Ocean area must prioritize finding and implementing a long-term solution to the problem of dwindling coastal fish stocks and rising human settlements along the coast.

3.2.3 Animals as a Source of Food

Large-scale livestock farming and related food chains are mainly meeting the rising demand for animal products in numerous nations across the world. Hundreds of millions of small-scale farmers and pastoralists, however, rely on animals to make a living. Aside from food production, farm animals serve a variety of purposes and services in the economy, culture, and society. They play an important role in agro-ecosystems.

Many foods that derive from an animal source, such as eggs, milk, meat, fish, honey, yogurt, and cheese, are considered animal source foods. Many people do not eat ASF or consume only a little amount of it due to personal preference or need, as ASF may not always be available or accessible to them. ASF is high in six micronutrients: vitamin A, vitamin B12, riboflavin (commonly known as vitamin B2), calcium, iron, and zinc. They play an important part in children's growth and development. Poor development, anemias (macrocytic anemia and iron deficiency anemia), bone disease, night blindness, impaired cognitive performance, neuromuscular deficiencies, diminished functional ability, psychiatric disorders, and death is all linked to insufficient stores of these micronutrients, which can be caused by either inadequate intake or poor absorption. Some of these consequences, such as decreased cognitive development caused by an iron deficit, are permanent (Shockley & Dossey, 2014).

Micronutrient insufficiency has been linked to delayed cognitive development in children. Infants, children, and pregnant women should be the focus of programs addressing micronutrient deficits. To address these major vitamin deficits, a snack program was created and tested in Kenyan schoolchildren by several global health experts and practitioners.

According to a report published by the United Nations in 2006, "the cattle industry sector appears as one of the top two or three most major contributors to the most significant environmental concerns, at all scales from local to global." As a result, eating plant-based meals is generally seen to be beneficial for the environment. Despite this, certain animals can be raised in a more ecologically friendly manner than others (Saberi et al., 2017). Raising rabbits and hens for food (on a well-considered method) can still be highly sustainable, according to a 1976 report from the Farralones Institute. As a result, meat and other products, such as eggs, may still be seen as ecologically beneficial (if this is done industrially with high efficiency).

Breeding goats (for goat meat and milk) may also be environmentally good, and some environmental advocates, such as Mahatma Gandhi, have advocated for it. The EAT-Lancet commission's global diet has recommended significant decreases in ASF consumption, claiming that these diets are unsustainable because of their ecological footprint and detrimental health effects. Adegbola T. Adesogan and colleagues challenged this report in 2020, claiming that it "failed to sufficiently include the encounter of marginalized children and women in low- and middle-income nations whose diets routinely lack the necessary nutrients," and that ASF is the best source of nutrient-rich food for children aged 6–23 months. Overcoming dietary quantity and quality inadequacies is a serious nutritional concern across the world, especially in impoverished nations. Diet quality is concerned with the capacity of the diet to supply high biologic value protein (existence of all essential amino acids) and sufficient amounts of micronutrients (i.e., minerals, vitamins, and trace metals) to achieve biological needs under a wide range of metabolic and environmental conditions, while diet quantity is concerned with the accessibility and intake of total food energy (kcal). Since the late 1980s, when the focus shifted to the energy gap, there has been a growing awareness of "hidden" malnutrition or multiple micronutrient deficiencies, as well as an understanding that diet quality is just as essential as diet quantity. Iron, calcium, iodine, zinc, vitamins A and B12, and, more recently, folate, are micronutrients of important significance in the development and growth, and health of children (Rochfort, 2005). Although many of them have significant economic and social consequences, only those that are most pertinent to animal-source foods are discussed in this section.

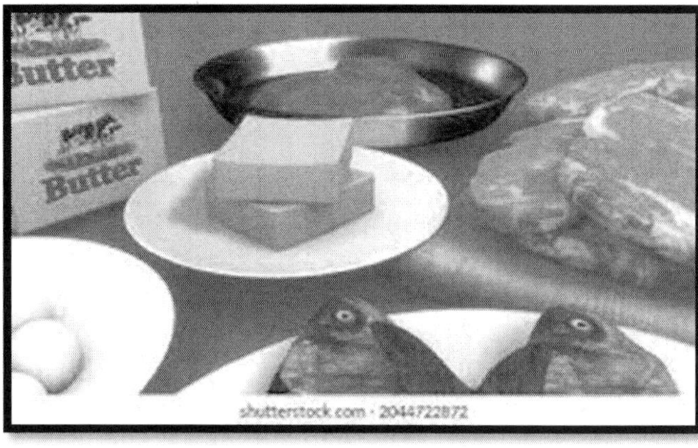

Figure 3.3: Animal source products.

Animal source meals are abundant in calories and a good source of high-quality, easily digestible protein. The proteins in these meals are of the greatest quality accessible since they include all of the necessary amino acids and are the most similar in amino acid composition to the proteins found in the human body. Animal-based meals are a good source of micronutrients as well. Iron, vitamin A, and zinc from meat, and vitamin B12, riboflavin, and calcium from milk are the key micronutrients given in ample and accessible form by animal source meals. Take a look at an example diet that includes maize and beans vs one that includes meat to see how beneficial adding micronutrient-dense meat to a child's diet may be (Ribeiro et al., 2019).

A youngster would need to ingest 1.7–2.0 kg of beans and maize in one day to fulfill the average daily needs for calories, iron, and zinc. This is significantly more than a youngster can handle, yet the same amount of meat might be consumed in 60 g (2 oz) every day. Similarly, dairy products are a significant source of calcium, and a child's typical calcium needs (estimated at 345 mg/d) are difficult to meet on a cereal-based diet. Riboflavin, selenium, taurine, and the long-chain polyunsaturated triglycerides, pentaenoic and hexaenoic acids, are all nutrients abundantly given by meat, chicken, and fish, and are all increasingly recognized as necessary for good human health. The fundamental benefit of animal source meals, particularly meat, is the high quantity and accessibility of micronutrients; that is, the presence of heme protein, which is present only in meat, fish, and fowl, allows for a high degree of absorption and assimilation by the body. Although some plant meals, such as spinach and legumes, are abundant in iron, zinc, or calcium, the micronutrients are inadequately absorbed. Leafy plants are high in oxalate, which forms insoluble compounds in the gut, reducing the number of minerals absorbed.

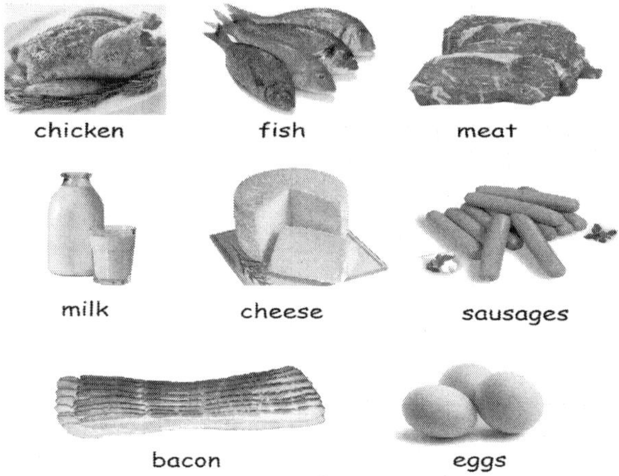

Figure 3.4: Meat is a source of energy, high-quality protein, and important vitamins (e.g., iron, zinc, vitamin A, vitamin B-12)

While there is proof that certain people should limit their intake of particular forms of ASF to enhance their health, the goal should be to achieve and maintain recommended daily intakes of several dietary categories, including ASF. To that aim, improving access to and consumption of modest amounts of ASF should be a worldwide priority for people living in locations where undernutrition is still an issue, especially for babies and women of childbearing age.

Unfortunately, the current focus on the detrimental effect of animal production has skewed this debate. By focusing on production systems that meet the ASF demand of high-income regions of the world and the negative consequences of excessive consumption there, international attention and dialogue miss the perspective and requirements of the large number of people living in low- and middle-income countries (LMICs), for whom improving ASF consumption could avert stunting and promote better health and development outcomes (Acosta-Estrada et al., 2021). The impact of low ASF consumption on the lives and futures of nutritionally vulnerable groups, women, and children, is a perspective that is generally omitted or underrepresented in scientific analysis or heated arguments on the effects of ASF production on climate change.

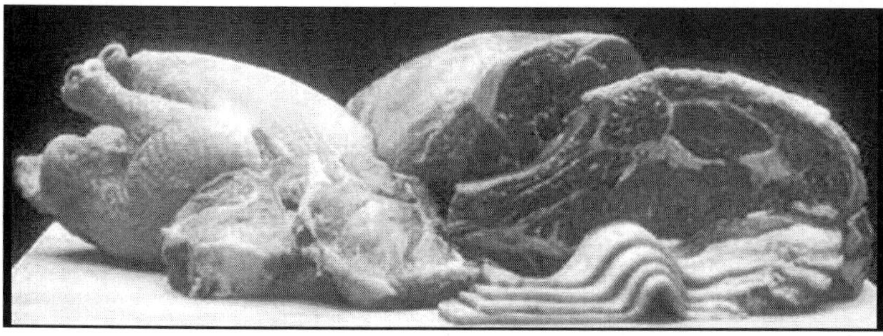

Figure 3.5: Animal by-products are products collected or generated from cattle that are not muscular meat, according to the USDA.

What's also absent is a grasp of how low ASF consumption is among the poor, especially in LMICs where starch-based diets are the norm. For example, in the worst four meat-consuming nations (Bangladesh, India, Sudan, and Ethiopia), the mean annual per capita meat consumption is less than one-third of that in the top four (USA, Australia, Uruguay, and Brazil). With rising per capita meat intake, there is a declining tendency in the number of stunted children in many nations throughout the world. While this association at the country level cannot be construed as proof of a causal relation, and while it may represent the income effect of certain ASF like meat, it supports the studies of Heady et al, Pimpin et al, and the supposition that ASF has advantageous impacts on child growth, which necessitates further assessment at the individual level in various settings (Reis *et al.,* 2017).

The United Nations issued a resolution in 2015 calling for the world to be transformed by 2030 by accomplishing 17 ambitious Sustainable Development Goals (SDGs). Poverty eradication, hunger eradication, excellent health and wellness, high-quality education, gender equality, decent employment and economic growth, inexpensive renewable energy, and climate action are just a few examples. Even though the goals are based on the previous Millennium Development Targets, they have been enhanced to include concrete goals and indicators for which poor nations must aspire. The new targets show that all nations have crucial work ahead of them if global sustainability is to be accomplished and that there are fundamental and significant disparities in the work that needs to be done.

It's worth noting that livestock is critical to achieving the SDGs, partially because they play such a significant role in the lives of the impoverished. LGA (2016) and FAO (2016) provided detailed explanations of the significance of livestock in attaining the SDGs (2018a). The following are some of the significant highlights: Without attention to the livestock industry, the world's fastest expanding agricultural sub-sector, which accounts for five of the ten highest value commodities in the world and 40 percent of global agricultural GDP in developing nations, poverty elimination is very improbable. Without livestock, improving food security and eradicating hunger would be far more difficult than it currently is for over 50% of the world's impoverished people, who depend on the sector for subsistence, income, insurance, and food (Raes et al., 2004). Furthermore, animal production permits food production in 57 percent of the earth's ecosystems that cannot be utilized for crop production, and livestock production provided 25% of protein and 18% of caloric intake globally in 2016, both of which are essential for nutritional security.

For around a third of farmers in underdeveloped nations, livestock supplied draught power or traction, however, a more recent estimate puts the figure at 50%. Livestock manure serves as organic fertilizer for more than half of the world's croplands, transforming waste products into high-value food inputs. Manure contributes to the replenishment of soil organic matter, which is essential for sustaining soil health and quality, as well as crop production and the restoration of damaged soils. By transforming millions of tons of agro-industrial by-products that cannot be eaten by people into livestock feeds, animal source food production helps significantly to the aims of a sustainable food system, decreasing waste and pollution while boosting human-consumable food. It's also worth noting that, according to recent FAO statistics, only around 14% of the feed dry matter eaten by livestock is edible to humans, and this proportion is likely significantly lower in numerous poor nations where ruminant animals eat mostly grasslands or crop wastes (Proksch *et al.*, 2003).

All livestock systems, like other farming production, contribute to environmental contamination in diverse ways and to variable degrees. To increase environmental stewardship, each livestock system should evaluate which of the aforementioned techniques it should use. In Sub-Saharan Africa and South Asia, livestock production is currently poor compared to their greenhouse gas emissions, resulting in greater greenhouse gas emission concentrations. For instance, to produce the same amount of milk as an average US dairy cow in a year (10,000 L), about 8 Indian dairy cows (producing a mean of 1200 L yearly) would be necessary, resulting in nine times the amount of methane generated from gastrointestinal sources.

Generally, Animal Sourced food is a very important aspect of our diets. Therefore, the "own production to consumption" pathway is one of the ways that agriculture initiatives, such as livestock transfers, might affect the intake of nutritious foods like ASFs and child nutritional status. This route is founded on the notion that home food production leads to ASF consumption, which leads to improved nutrient intake and excellent nutritional outcomes, particularly for children (Pop *et al.,* 2019). Social and behavior change communication (SBCC), which includes group sessions, home visits, town hall meetings, and mass media, can impact and improve food production, expenditures, and consumption. In families where SBCC is introduced into livestock production treatments, children's consumption of ASFs and, as a result, their nutritional condition improves.

3.2.4 Crop Cultivation as a Food Source

The grass family (Poaceae) is the fifth biggest flowering plant family in the world, but it is the most vital for humans. 3/5 of all human calories are provided by three grass species (maize, rice, and wheat). These three species, along with 17 cultivars, account for 85 percent of all calories consumed on the planet. Plant foods are good suppliers of nutrition and energy, but humans eat them for a variety of reasons. In almost all societies, food crops have symbolic and ceremonial significance. Due to the abundance of allelochemical substances found in many food species, they offer therapeutic benefits. Not all of these chemicals are good for you. Plant foods are detoxified by humans via biological, behavioral, and technological methods before they are ingested (Ambuja & Rajakumar, 2018).

Plants are an inexhaustible source of sustenance for humans. Many plant-derived medications, textiles, and colors can be replaced with synthetic chemicals and petroleum derivatives; metal, brick, and concrete may be used to replace wood; but there is no equivalent for plant-derived foods. Plants or creatures that consume plants account for nearly all human diets. Saprophytic fungus makes up a small percentage of most people's daily calorie intake. As previously said, the early people gathered wild species.

High-yielding cultivars are used in modern societies to provide them with more control over food supplies. While hunger and food shortages continue to be problems in some regions of the world, more than 90% of the world's population lives in some places (for example, Sub-Saharan Africa and the Indian subcontinent) with consistent and sufficient food supply. Many anthropologists believe that increasing food supply management has been the most crucial element in human society's evolution (Odhaib et al., 2021). Food crop yield, palatability, and nutritional value have all enhanced as a result of recent genetic alterations of cultivars. Nonetheless, traditional farmers cultivated all of the world's food plants between 9,000 and 10,000 years ago. This chapter discusses the major food crops and the benefits of eating plant foods, as well as a quick summary of food toxicity.

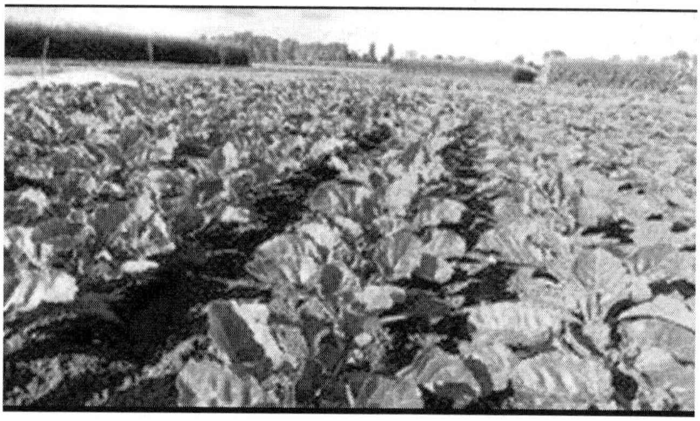

Figure 3.6: Cultivation.

Only three grasses – rice (*Oryza sativa*), maize (*Zea mays*), and wheat (*Triticum aestivum*) – provide 85 percent of human calories, whereas 20 plant species provide 60 percent (*Zea mays*). Only a few hundred vascular plants have been domesticated, and only around 1% of the world's vascular plants have been major food sources. Surprisingly, none of these twenty essential foods can be traced back to contemporary agriculture. Traditional farmers developed all of them between 2,000 and 9,000 years ago. Our original subsistence strategy was foraging for wild plant and animal resources. Despite the existence of a few foraging or pastoralist societies, the majority of the world's population depends on cultivated species to meet their daily nutritional demands.

The grass family contains the four most frequently grown species on the planet. Sugar cane (*Saccharum officinarum*) is grown in greater quantities than any other cultivated grass, yet only a small portion of it is consumed directly. Sugar cane is a key source of table sugar and is also used to make ethanol. Similar methods are utilized with sugar beets, which rank sixth in yearly yield. Due to rising ethanol demand, maize (or corn) output has surged in recent years (Murdoch *et al*., 2000).

Obtaining nourishment and energy is the obvious option as to why food is important. Plants offer the majority of daily calories and roughly 65 percent of protein in all but a few modern societies. Growing archaeological evidence reveals that Paleolithic people's diets were not as meat-centric as previously thought. Plant foods most likely made-up half or more of their diets. While nutritional and energy demands for growth, development, and equilibrium are important, they are not the sole reasons to consume meals. The line between food and medicine is blurry in many cultures. Foods supply calories and nutrition, but they also include a variety of chemical substances that can help to prevent or treat disease. Foods and meals have tremendous ceremonial and symbolic significance. Floodways, like language and religion, are one of the distinguishing characteristics of a civilization.

Fruits and vegetables are essential components of every diet, not just for vegetarians but also for non-vegetarians. They are plant derivatives that are typically developed in ovaries, fruits, flowers, stems, and leaves. Vitamins and minerals may be found in abundance in fruits and vegetables. Fresh fruits and vegetables, juices, and salads are major sources of crucial minerals and vitamins these days, and they are being emphasized more than ever. Heart disease, cancer, metabolic disorders, nutritional anemia, and other illnesses can all be prevented by eating a diet rich in fruits and vegetables, according to epidemiological research. Low plasma levels of antioxidant micronutrients, which are often present in fruits and vegetables, are linked to an increased risk of several illnesses.

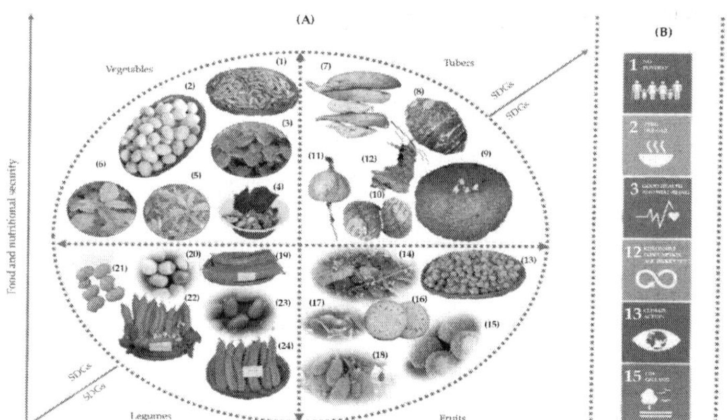

Figure 3.7: Food crops.

(Source: Singh A, Dubey PK, et, al., 2019)

Because many of the plants we raise for sustenance are not fully domesticated, the term "crop" is wide and vague, which is probably fitting because the phrase encompasses all that is harvested regardless of its status as a domesticate. As a result, we must draw as clear a distinction as possible between farmed and domesticated animals (Multari *et al.*, 2015). Although the names are frequently used interchangeably, they have quite distinct meanings. The term "domesticate" refers to the act of bringing something into one's home. Domesticated plants and animals are those that have been genetically transformed from their natural condition and have adapted to live with humans.

Because domestication is an evolutionary process, all degrees of plant and animal interaction with humans will be found, as well as a variety of physical divergence, ranging from races that are identical to those found in the wild to fully domesticated races. For survival, a fully domesticated plant or animal is wholly reliant on humans. As a result, domestication entails a shift in ecological adaptability, which is typically linked to morphological differences. Many transitional phases are unavoidable. Tilling the soil, establishing a seedbed, weeding, trimming, protecting, watering, and manuring are all examples of actions that go into caring for a plant. Domestication is concerned with the genetic response of the animals or plants being cared for or cultivated, whereas cultivation is focused on human activity. Wild species can therefore be grown, while cultivated plants do not always have to be domesticated.

By focusing on the protein crisis, we can concentrate our emphasis on the global food situation. To begin with, the human body does not require protein; rather, it requires a supply of critical amino acids that the body cannot make. By boosting the nutritional benefits of the proteins generated, we may help to improve the protein situation. The most prevalent protein quality inadequacies in cereals are lysine, methionine, and tryptophan. Threonine deficiency is also common in rice. In certain circumstances, there are just minor shortages (Lin et al., 2010). For example, high-quality high-protein wheat is a rich source of dietary protein. The limiting amino acid is lysine, yet there is enough of it to keep life and health going.

However, lysine levels in maize are so low that significant malnutrition symptoms, particularly in children, can emerge. Kwashiorkor is a dietary disorder induced by a lack of lysine in the context of a low protein diet. If humans stopped feeding protein-rich foods to animals, there would be a lot more protein available. Even though the United States produces 70% of the world's soybeans, just around 2% of them are consumed directly by people. Almost all of it is processed and used to feed chickens, pigs, and cattle.

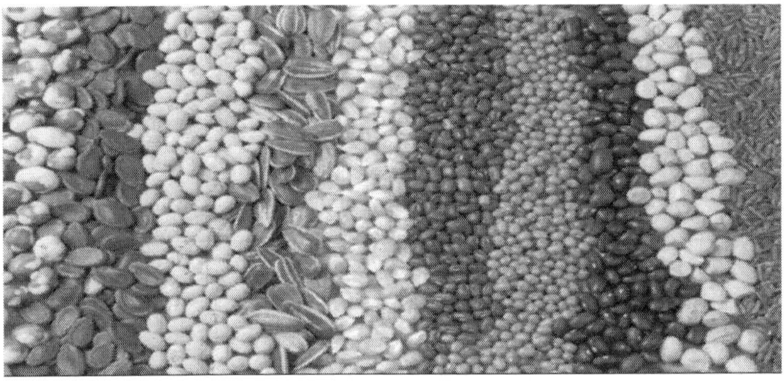

Figure 3.8: Grains dried beans and legumes.

The animals are subsequently ingested, and while animal protein is superior to vegetable protein in terms of quality, the conversion wastes overall protein in human meals. North Americans will most likely consume less meat in the future, and this moment has already arrived for the majority of the world's population. Plants provide almost 80% of the protein in the human diet in Asia and Africa, while animal sources provide around 20%. Animal sources account for over 70% of the protein in developed portions of North America, while vegetables account for barely 30%. Changes in these ratios may be forced by population pressures (Ananda et al., 2017).

In fact, certain populations depend on plants only as their only source of food. All animal products, including meat, dairy, and eggs, are prohibited in a vegan or plant-based diet. Vegan diets may be very nutritious, minimize the risk of chronic illnesses, and promote weight reduction when followed correctly. Vegan diets are becoming more popular as people become more concerned about their health, animal welfare, and the environment. According to a Gallup study conducted in 2018, roughly 3% of Americans are entirely vegan, and sales of plant-based products are increasing. Vegan diets are nutrient-dense and low in saturated fats. According to research, eating a healthy diet can enhance heart health, prevent cancer, and reduce the incidence of type 2 diabetes. People who consume purely plant-based foods, on the other hand, should be more cognizant of how to get certain minerals, such as iron, calcium, and vitamin B-12, which are often found in an omnivorous diet.

A vegan diet consists only of plant-based meals. All animal products, including meat, dairy, and eggs, are avoided by those who follow this diet. Honey is also avoided by some folks. Veganism is a nutritional choice for some, but it is also a lifestyle decision for others. Vegans avoid wearing garments, soaps, and other things that utilize or include animal components, such as leather and animal hair. Some people choose this lifestyle as a sustainable diet because of its environmental benefits. Fruits, vegetables, legumes, nuts, and seeds are commonly found in vegan diets. A wide range of critical vitamins, minerals, healthy fats, and protein may be obtained by eating a variety of these foods (Linares *et al.,* 2017).

Plants contain critical elements that are unavailable from other sources. Plants include vitamins, minerals, phytochemicals, and antioxidants that help maintain your cells healthy and your body in balance, allowing your immune system to perform at its best. Plants provide your body with the nutrients it requires to fight illness. Your immune system is strengthened by a plant-based diet, which protects you from germs and pathogens. Because it can spot and target abnormalities in cells before they proceed to illness, a functioning immune system is critical for lowering your cancer risk.

Inflammation is reduced by eating plant foods. The vital nutrients included in plants help to reduce inflammation in the body. The same phytochemicals and antioxidants that enhance your immune system also neutralize poisons from pollution, processed foods, germs, viruses, and other sources throughout your body. Plant antioxidants scavenge all of the so-called free radicals that might upset your body's equilibrium. To minimize inflammation, eat a plant-based diet and pay attention to your body's messages about how foods affect you. Prolonged inflammation has been related to cancer and other inflammatory conditions like arthritis, and it can harm your body's cells and tissue. Because it eliminates some of the illnesses' causes, a plant-based diet may protect you (López *et al*., 2019).

Maintaining a healthy weight is easier with a plant-based diet. One of the most essential things you can do to lower your cancer risk is to maintain a healthy weight. The only thing more essential than keeping a healthy weight when it comes to cancer prevention is not smoking. This is since being overweight induces inflammation as well as hormone imbalances. If you are overweight or obese, you are more likely to get colorectal, postmenopausal breast, pancreatic, kidney, esophageal, and uterine cancers, to name a few. Many of the things that cause weight gain are eliminated when you eat largely vegetables. When you add exercise to the mix, you're on your way to losing weight. Fiber is abundant in plants. All unprocessed plant foods include fiber. It is what gives the plant its structure, and eating more of it gives you access to a slew of advantages. Eating a plant-based diet enhances gut health, allowing you to absorb more nutrients from the food that help your immune system and reduce inflammatory processes. Fiber can help decrease cholesterol and blood sugar levels, and it's also beneficial for intestinal health. Fiber is crucial in lowering your cancer risk. This is especially true if you are at risk for colorectal cancer, the third most prevalent malignancy.

A plant-based diet also lowers your chances of contracting other ailments. The advantages of eating primarily vegetables go beyond lowering your cancer risk. A plant-based diet has also been demonstrated to lower the risk of heart disease, stroke, hypertension, and some mental diseases.

Even a plant-based dinner depends on you to stay away from common dietary hazards like sugar and fat. Using good cooking methods and understanding how to maximize the nutritional value of your veggies will help you reap the full advantages of a plant-based diet. Deep-fried veggies are no longer an option (Karioti et al., 2015). Highly processed meals, such as crackers and cookies, are also unhealthy. Limit sugary treats as well, and choose whole grains if possible. Although regular pasta, white bread, and white rice are all plant-based, they are not prepared from whole grains. Eat brown rice and 100 percent whole wheat pasta and toast. Plants will assist all of your body's systems in performing at their best.

3.3 CONCLUSION

Food systems throughout the world may brag about their accomplishments. The world population more than quadrupled between 1960 and now, yet global food production tripled, assuring more food per person at cheaper prices. Furthermore, by increasing production per unit of agricultural land, food systems were able to do this while only needing roughly 10-15% additional agricultural area. The growth of agricultural land has had a significant detrimental impact on forests and biodiversity, as well as a significant increase in greenhouse gas emissions. The ramifications for environmental and human well-being would have been disastrous if food systems had not been able to enhance output.

Reforming policies relating to food systems has proven to be difficult in the past. It has demonstrated that improving policies necessitate resolving conflicts over facts, goals, and values. Although much is known about which policy changes might help food systems, there are still considerable information gaps concerning the scope and nature of issues, synergies and trade-offs, and the benefits and costs of various policy alternatives for many policy challenges. There may also be discrepancies between public opinions and scientific data, and policy debates may be impeded by misconceptions, misunderstandings, or obsolete perspectives (Khorram & Ramezanian, 2021). However, facts aren't the main source of disagreement in the policymaking process. This being said, with all that we have discussed regarding food sources, there is a whole need for policy-driven initiatives to provide adequate and required food sources all over the world.

CHAPTER 4

UTILIZATION OF FOOD BY THE BODY

CONTENTS

Once food has been consumed, it is transformed into various formed and used in the body. Among the ways food is utilized in the body is as energy. All parts of the body need the energy to work. The energy is synthesized from the food we eat. When food is eaten it is digested by mixing with various fluids such as enzymes and acids in the stomach. During the digestion of food in the stomach, the carbohydrates such as starches and sugars are broken down into sugar known as glucose. The generated glucose is then absorbed by the stomach and small intestines. It eventually finds its way into the bloodstream. While in the bloodstream, glucose can readily be used as energy or stored in the body for later use (Karthika & Sureshkumar, 2021). Depending on the type of food, its utilization in the body is different. Carbohydrates are used in energy production that facilitates the working of various body parts, proteins are used in bodybuilding and repair of worn-out tissues while vitamins are used in protecting the body from diseases.

4.1 UTILIZATION OF CARBOHYDRATES IN THE BODY

Carbohydrates are also known as carbs are sugar molecules. Carbohydrates, fats, and proteins are among the main nutrients found in drinks and food. After carbohydrates are ingested, they are broken down into glucose. Glucose is at times known as blood sugar and is considered the main source of energy in body organs, tissues, and cells. Glucose is usually stored in the liver for future use and can also be used immediately by body muscles (Karwowska *et al.*, 2021). There are different kinds of carbohydrates each used differently by the body. The first type of carbohydrate is sugar. Sugars are also known as simple carbohydrates as they are in basic form. Simple sugars can be added to various food. For instance, sugar can be added to foods such as regular soda, processed foods, desserts, and candy. Some sugars are naturally found in milk, vegetables, and fruits.

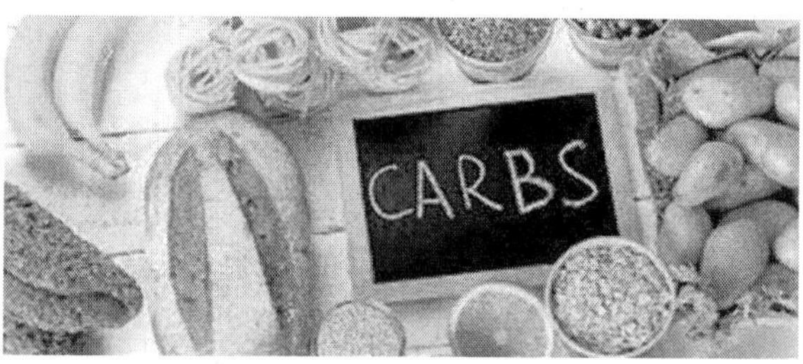

Figure 4.1: Carbohydrates are utilized as glucose in the body.

Starches are also part of carbohydrates. Starches are made of a large number of simple sugars that have been strung together. For starch to be used by the body, it has to be broken down into sugars used in energy production. Some examples of starches are pasta, cereal, bread, corn, peas, and potatoes. Another type of carbohydrate is fiber. They are a very complex form of carbohydrates. Usually, fibers cannot be broken down by the body. By eating large amounts of fiber, the body feels full and renders the person less likely to eat. Large amounts of fiber in the diet have significant health benefits. Fibers are useful in preventing intestinal or stomach problems such as constipation. Fibers are useful in lowering blood sugar and cholesterol level. Fiber is richly found in plants such as whole grains, beans, seeds, nuts, vegetables, and fruits (Kau *et al.,* 2011).

There are various foods rich in carbohydrates. They include grains such as rice, crackers, pasta, noodles, bread, and cereals. In fruits such as oranges, melons, mangoes, berries, bananas, and apples. In dairy products such as yogurt and milk, legumes such as peas, lentils, and dried beans, snack foods and sweets such as desserts, candy, cookies, and cakes, starchy vegetables such as peas, corn, and potatoes, and also in juices, fruit drinks, regular sodas, sports drinks and energy drinks with sugar. Some foods have carbohydrates but in small amounts. They include nuts, cheese, oils, poultry, fish, and meat

All the different kinds of carbohydrates are utilized in the body in different ways. There are five main uses of carbohydrates in the human body. The uses include assisting lipid metabolism, sparing protein, building macromolecules, energy storage, and energy production.

4.2 ENERGY PRODUCTION

Under energy production, carbohydrates are useful in supplying energy to all cells in the body. It was noted that cells have a preference for glucose as a source of energy compared to other compounds such as fatty acids. Red blood cells are examples of cells with the ability to produce cellular energy from glucose. Our brains are naturally sensitive to low blood glucose levels. This is explained by the fact that the brain uses glucose in energy production and function. This is in exception of situations where there are extreme starvation conditions.

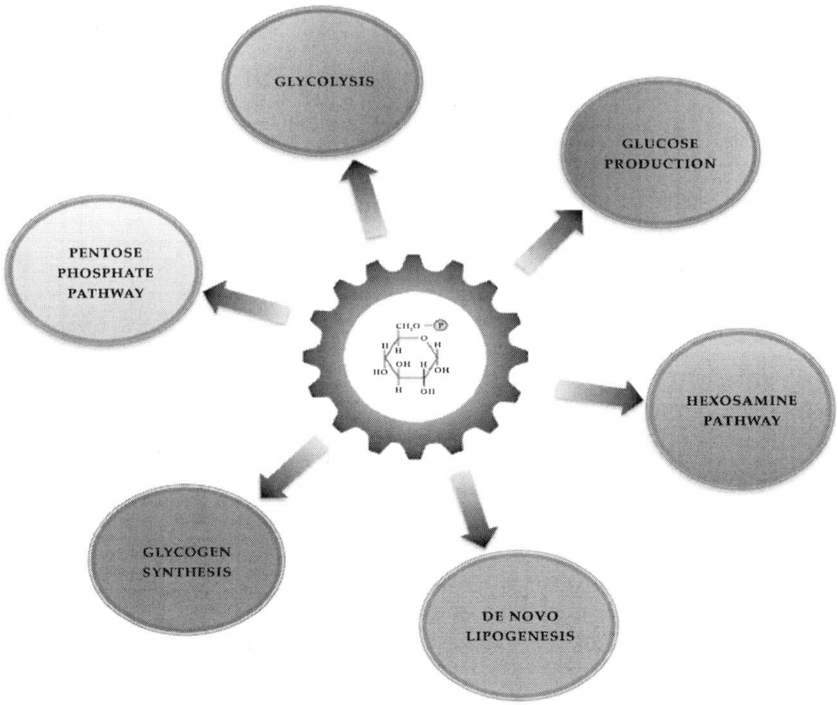

Figure 4.2: Carbohydrates are used to provide the energy needed by the body.

(Source: Rajas F, Gautier-Stein A, et, al., 2019).

The total amount of glucose entering the body through digestion, about 70% is redistributed by the liver into the blood for use by other tissues. Cells need the energy to remove glucose from blood with a transport protein in their membranes. Energy used by these cells is gotten from chemical bonds between carbon atoms. A process known as photosynthesis makes use of sunlight when producing high-energy bonds. Our body cells then break the chemical bonds and also capture energy needed in cellular respiration. Cellular respiration is a process that involves a controlled burning of glucose versus an uncontrolled burning. Cells are known to use several chemical reactions in several enzymatic steps to slow down the release of energy to prevent an explosion and efficiently capture energy preserved within the chemical bonds in glucose (Kadam & Prabhasankar, 2010).

The first step of cellular respiration is the breaking down of glucose known as glycolysis. Glycolysis is also known as the splitting of glucose. This process occurs in intricate series of ten enzymatic-reaction steps. The second stage of the breakdown of glucose occurs in the energy factory organelles neon as mitochondria. The process involves the removal of one carbon atom and two oxygen atoms resulting in more energy. Energy from the carbon bonds is carried to an area known as the mitochondria. This makes cellular energy available in a form that can be used by cells. The utilization of carbohydrates in the body mostly involves the mitochondria.

There are various roles of mitochondria in food utilization. The main goal of degradation of foodstuffs is the conversion of energy contained in chemical bonds on the energy-rich compound adenosine triphosphate. The compound is used in capturing chemical energy obtained from the breakdown of food molecules while releasing its fuels in other cellular processes. Eukaryotic cells are those organisms that possess a clear definition of the nucleus and membrane-bound organelles. In eukaryotic cells, enzymes needed in the catalyzation of individual steps involved in energy and respiration conservation are located in highly organized rod-shaped compartments known as mitochondria. In microorganisms, useful enzymes occur as components of the cell membrane. In the liver, there are about 1,000 mitochondria while large egg cells of some vertebrates have about 200,000.

The utilization of food is also covered by the Tricarboxylic acid cycle. This cycle is also known as the citric acid cycle or the Krebs cycle. They play an important role in the breakdown or catabolism of organic fuel molecules. This cycle consists of eight steps catalyzed by eight different enzymes involved in energy production at different stages. Large amounts of energy obtained from the cycle are captured by compounds flavin adenine dinucleotide and NAD+. It is later on converted into ATP. A single turn of the TCA cycle is made up of three NAD+ molecules that are reduced through the addition of hydrogen (Jacob et al., 2020). Reduction is done to the same number of NADH molecules and a single FAD molecule. It is then further reduced into a single FADH2 molecule. The molecules proceed to fuel the third stage of cellular respiration. The waste product of the cycle is carbon dioxide.

Another stage is oxidative phosphorylation which involves each pair of hydrogen atoms being removed from FADH2 and NADH. They provide a pair of electrons through the action of a series of iron-containing hemoproteins. The reduction of one atom of oxygen to form water is done by cytochromes. It was discovered that the transfer of one pair of electrons to oxygen results in three molecules of ATP being formed. Oxidative phosphorylation is said to be a major mechanism through which large amounts of energy in foodstuffs are conserved and made available to cells. There are several steps through which electrons flow to oxygen allowing the gradual lowering of energy of electrons. This stage is known as the electron transport chain. Some have renamed this stage in cellular respiration the electron transport chain.

The theoretical yield of ATP molecules per glucose during cellular respiration is 38. However, these conditions are often not realized due to losses such as the cost of moving private from glycolysis and ADP into the mitochondria. Carriers are usually involved in the active transportation that uses the stored energy in the proton electrochemical gradient. During this stage, pyruvate is taken up by a low Km transporter bringing it into the mitochondrial matrix for oxidation by the pyruvate dehydrogenase complex. The phosphate carrier is useful in mediating the electroneutral exchange of phosphate for OH-. It also involves the symport of phosphate and protons across the inner membrane (Ibrahim *et al.*, 2015). The proton motive force is the driving force for moving phosphate ions into the mitochondria. The adenine nucleotide translocase also called the ATP-ADP translocase is an antiporter. It is involved in the exchange of ATP and ADO across the inner membrane. The driving force is brought about by ATP having a more negative charge compared to the ADP. It is involved in the dissipation of certain electrical components in the proton electrochemical gradient.

Transportation while utilizing the proton electrochemical gradient produces more than 3 H+ all needed in making 1ATP. This, therefore, reduces the theoretical efficiency of the entire process. The maximum is closer to 28-39 ATP molecules. In a practice scenario, the efficiency may be lower as the inner membrane of mitochondria may be leaky to protons. Other factors may lead to the dissipation of the proton gradient leading to leaky mitochondria. Thermogenin is an uncoupling protein that is expressed in some cell types. It is at times used as a channel that can transport protons. When thermogenin is active in the inner membrane it short circuits the coupling between the ATP synthesis and electron transport chain. It is important to note that the potential energy from the proton gradient is used in heat generation rather than the creation of ATP. The generation of heat is very important in the brown fat thermogenesis of newborns and hibernating mammals. Cellular respiration is a process that facilitates the oxidation of biological fuels in the presence of high-energy inorganic electron acceptors like oxygen in the production of large amounts of energy. They drive the bulk production of ATP (Hou & Xu, 2022).

Food is used in energy production in the body through anaerobic respiration. This kind of energy production is done when the body is experiencing a deficit of energy. This kind of energy production involves the use of an inorganic acceptor such as sulfur, nitrate, and sulfate. This kind of energy production is mostly exhibited in athletes when they take part in extensively long races which may cause them to take in small amounts of oxygen.

4.3 ENERGY STORAGE

Carbohydrates are greatly used in energy storage. There are instances where the body needs energy but there are no ready sources of energy. For this reason, the stored energy is used. Here are cases where the body would get enough energy to support its functions and the excess glucose is stored as glycogen. Glycogen is mostly stored in the liver and muscles. A single molecule of glycogen may have an excess of fifty thousand single glucose units. It is usually highly branched to facilitate the rapid dissemination of glucose when there is a need for cellular energy.

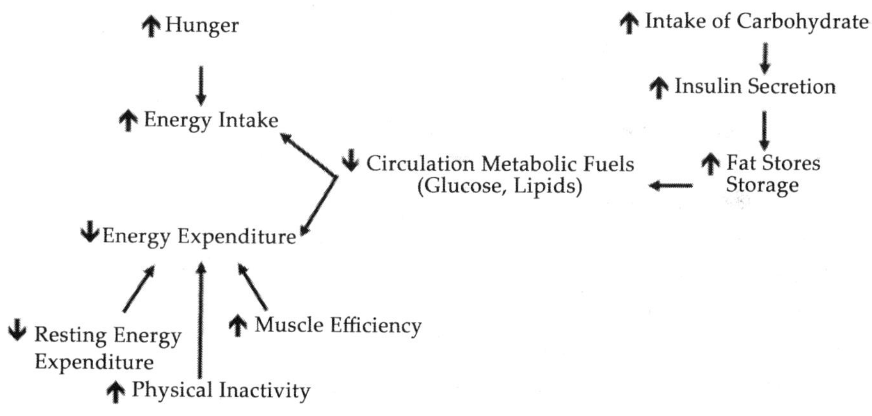

Figure 4.3: Carbohydrates can be stored to enable the provision of energy in the absence of food.

(Source: Seid H, and Rosenbaum M. 2019)

At any one time, the amount of glycogen in the body is equivalent to about 4,000 kilocalories to 3,000 in muscle tissue and 1,000 in the liver. When the muscles are used for relatively long durations of time, the glycogen energy reserve can be depleted. This kind of energy depletion is referred to as bonking or hitting the wall. This condition is characterized by fatigue and also a decrease in exercise performance. When the muscles weaken, it takes longer amounts of time to transform the chemical energy in fatty acids and proteins into usable energy than glucose. Prolonged exercise durations cause glycogen depletion and the muscles may need to rely more on proteins and lipids as a source of energy. To increase the glycogen reserve, athletes may reduce their training intensity while increasing the number of carbohydrates they consume to between 60-70% of the total calories three to five days before an event (Haque *et al.*, 2020). For people who do not do hardcore training and choose to run a 5-kilometer race for fun may not need to take a big plate of pasta before a race as without long-term intense training the adaptation of increased muscle glycogen may not happen.

The muscles of the body and the liver can store energy as glycogen. However, when compared to the muscle tissue the liver will sacrifice its stored glucose energy to other tissues in the body when there are low levels of glucose in the blood. About one-quarter of the total body glycogen content is in the liver and is equivalent to about a four-hour supply of glucose. This is highly dependent on the level of activity. The glycogen reserve in the liver is used in keeping blood glucose levels within a narrow range between meal times. When glycogen supply in the liver is exhausted, glucose is made from amino acids from the destruction of proteins to maintain metabolic homeostasis.

4.4 BUILDING MACROMOLECULES

In the total amounts of glucose in the body, a large amount of glucose is used in making energy while the rest is converted to ribose and deoxyribose which are essential in buildings blocks of important macromolecules such as ATP, DNA, and RNA. Glucose is also used in making the molecule NADPH which is very useful in protecting the body against oxidative stress and is utilized in other chemical reactions in the body. When all the energy needs in the body are met, excess glucose is used in making fat. This is why the addition of large amounts of carbon in the diet and calories could add on the fat pounds (Halloran *et al.*, 2015).

4.5 SPARING PROTEIN

There are cases where the amount of glucose in the body is not enough to meet the body's demands. For this reason, the needed oxygen is synthesized from amino acids. Usually, there is no storage molecule for amino acids.

The process of making energy may require the destruction of protein more so from the muscle tissue. When there are sufficient amounts of glucose in the body then there is no need for the breakdown of proteins from being used to generate glucose for the body.

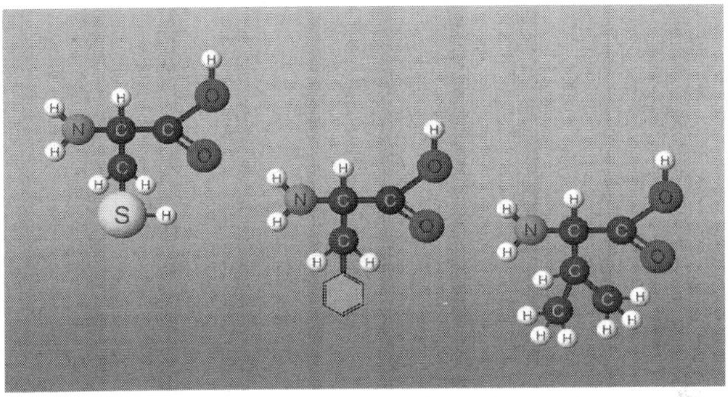

Figure 4.4: Amino acids can be used to create the energy needed in the body.

4.6 LIPID METABOLISM

The use of lipids as a source of energy is inhibited by the level of blood glucose levels. Glucose is said to have a fat-sparing effect. This is explained by the fact that an increase in blood glucose stimulates the release of insulin that tells cells to make use of glucose rather than lipids in making energy. Sufficient amounts of glucose in the blood are useful in preventing the development of ketosis. Ketosis is defined as a metabolic condition caused by an elevation of ketone bodies in the blood. The ketone body can be used as an alternative source of energy that can be used by cells when there are insufficient amounts of glucose similar to fasting. By nature, the ketone bodies are acidic. If present in the blood in large amounts can cause it to become very acidic. Such an occurrence is very rare in healthy adults but is a frequent occurrence in alcoholics, people with Type1 diabetes, and malnourished individuals. To inhibit ketosis in adults, the minimum amount of carbohydrates needed is 50 grams per day (Hathwar et al., 2012). The utilization of carbohydrates in the body is useful in supporting life's basic function through the production of energy. The absence of energy would mean that none of these processes could be possible. Glucose synthesis comes at the cost of protein destruction. However, consumption of carbohydrates should be done in moderation to avoid having too much or too little in the diet to avoid health problems.

The utilization of carbohydrates more so sugar is highly dependent on the production of insulin. Insulin is a hormone made by beta cells in the pancreas. By nature, the beta cells are usually very sensitive to the amount of glucose in the bloodstream. These cells usually check the amount of blood glucose levels every few seconds and sense whether they need to slow down or speed up the amount of insulin they are making and releasing. When food with large amounts of carbohydrates is consumed such as a piece of bread, the level of glucose in the blood increases triggering the pancreas to release more insulin into the bloodstream. Once the pancreas releases insulin, it travels through the bloodstream to the body's cells. It tells the cell doors to open allowing glucose in. When inside it, cells convert glucose into energy for use right then or store it for later use. The movement of glucose into cells causes blood sugar levels to start dropping (Ferreira & Nunes, 2019). As this occurs, the beta cells in the pancreas can detect that this is happening and as a response, they slow down the amount of insulin they are making. While this is going on, the pancreas slows down the amount of insulin g being released into the bloodstream. At the same time, the amount of glucose going into the cells slows down.

Fluctuations in the amount of insulin in blood sugar occur many times during the day and night. The amounts of insulin and glucose in the bloodstream are dependent on the amount of food consumed and when it was consumed. When the body is actively engaged such as during work hours, blood sugar is maintained in the target range which is between 70 and 140 milligrams per deciliter. However, there are cases when the level of blood sugar can rise to 180 right after a meal or during the meal. After two hours of eating, blood sugar levels are expected to drop to under 140. Several hours after eating, blood sugar can drop to as low as 70 (Francesconi, 2007).

Our bodies work by using glucose for energy and keeping it balanced with the right amounts of insulin. Maintaining the amount of energy ensures its survival as it takes part in various functions. To ensure the body can survive events without eating, the body stores extra glucose. Insulin is very useful in helping cells convert glucose into energy. It is also useful in storing the extra glucose for later use. This mostly happens when an individual consumes large amounts of food but the body does not need much glucose at the moment. Insulin will be involved in converting energy later. This is done by insulin turning the extra food into large packets of glucose called glycogen. Glycogen is usually stored in the muscles and liver. Insulin is so used in fat and protein storage. Proteins are key elements in the body as it enables the body to work and grow. The generated fat is used by the body in protecting the nerves and making several important hormones. Fats can also be used as an energy source when the individual has not eaten.

4.7 UTILIZATION OF FIBER IN THE BODY

Fiber form part of the kind of carbohydrate which cannot be digested by the body. Fiber is the only type of carbohydrate that cannot be broken down into sugar molecules. As it is not digested, fiber passes through the body undigested. Fiber is very useful in the body. It is involved in the regulation of the body's use of sugar. It helps keep hunger and blood sugar in check. Both adults and children require about 20 to 39 grams of fiber in a day for good health. Americans, their bodies get about 15 grams of fiber in a day (Fabani *et al.*, 2013). There are various sources of fiber in the body. They include beans, whole grains, vegetables, and fruits. There are two varieties of fibers that are beneficial to human health. The first kind is soluble fiber. This kind of fiber dissolves in water and is useful in lowering levels of glucose in the body. It is also used in lowering the amount of cholesterol. Examples of foods that contain soluble fiber include blueberries, apples, lentils, beans, nuts, and oatmeal. There is an insoluble fiber that does not dissolve in water. This kind of fiber is useful in helping food move through the digestive system and promotes regularity while preventing constipation. Examples of food with insoluble fibers include tomatoes, cucumbers, carrots, legumes, brown rice, whole grain couscous, whole wheat bread, and wheat. Sources considered the best sources of fiber include nuts, legumes, vegetables, fresh fruits, and whole grains. To increase the amount of fiber in the diet, individuals are advised to eat whole fruits rather than drinking fruit juices, replace white rice, pasta, and bread with whole grain products and brown rice, choose a cereal with whole grains for breakfast, snacking on raw vegetables rather than chocolate bars, crackers or chips and finally substituting legumes or beans for meat two to three times per week in soups and chili (Dixon & Sumner, 2003).

Fiber is greatly used by the body in reducing the risk of developing various conditions such as constipation, diverticular disease, diabetes, and heart disease. There is little knowledge to prove that fiber has effects on the risk of colon cancer. Under heart disease, consumption of large amounts of fiber had been linked to reduced risk of heart disease. A study done at Harvard on over 40,000 male health professionals showed that a high total dietary fiber intake was linked to a 40% reduced risk of coronary heart disease. A similar study was done among female nurses and produced similar findings. Consumption of fiber has been linked to reduced risks of metabolic syndrome, a combination of factors that increases the risk of development of diabetes and heart disease. Examples of these factors include low levels of HDL cholesterol, high levels of triglycerides, excess weight, high insulin levels and high blood pressure.

Various studies have been used to prove that the consumption of large amounts of fiber may offer protective benefits from the syndrome. When a diet is low in fiber but rich in food increases the likelihood of high blood sugar increases the body's ability to develop type 2 diabetes. Both studies done at Harvard covering both male and female health professionals led to the establishment that type 2 diabetes more than doubled the risk of type 2 diabetes when compared to a diet which high amounts of fiber in the diet and low high-glycemic-index foods (Da Silva *et al*., 2016). Lower risks of type 2 diabetes have been linked to high amounts of fiber in cereals. Fiber had also been useful in dealing with diverticular disease. This kind of disease is characterized by an inflammation of the intestine. It is considered among the common age-related disorders of the colon. A study done among male health professionals in a long-term follow-up study who were in dietary fiber more so insoluble fiber showed a reduced risk of diverticular disease.

Fiber is useful in preventing problems such as constipation. Constipation is said to be the most common gastrointestinal complaint in the United States. It was noted that the consumption of fiber is useful in relieving and preventing constipation. The amount of fiber in oat bran and wheat bran is more effective compared to fiber found in fruits and vegetables. For this reason, experts recommend increased consumption of the amount of fiber gradually rather than suddenly. Fiber is known to absorb water. For this reason, experts recommend that the intake of beverages should be increased with an increase in the amount of fiber consumed. Some suggest that fiber could be used in dealing with colon cancer. Studies done have failed to demonstrate the link between colon cancer and fiber. In the study, it was found that fiber is not strongly associated with a reduced risk for polyps and colon cancer (Dayan *et al.,* 2009). Incorporation of sufficient amounts of fiber in the diet has been linked to reduced risks of breast cancer. Studies done have been useful in suggesting that fiber intake during adolescence and early adulthood may be very important. It was noted that women who consume large amounts of fiber during adolescence and young adulthood have lower risks of breast cancer compared to those who take smaller amounts of dietary fiber when young.

4.8 UTILIZATION OF PROTEINS

Proteins are defined as macromolecules and biomolecules comprising one or more long chains of amino acid residues. Within the body, proteins perform different kinds of functions such as the provision of structure to cells and organisms, DNA replication, catalyzing metabolic reactions, and the transportation of molecules from one location to another. There are different kinds of proteins with the difference being brought by the sequence of amino acids that is dictated by the nucleotide sequence of genes that results in proteins folding into a particular 3D structure which determines its activity.

Proteins are actively involved in cellular functions. They are considered the chief actors in a cell as they carry out the duties specified by the information encoded in genes. RNA is very different from other biological molecules that are relatively inert elements acted upon by proteins. In an *Escherichia coli* cell, proteins make up about half the dry weight. Other components include RNA and DNA which make about 20% and 3% respectively (Caporgno & Mathys, 2018). The proteome is the set of proteins expressed in a particular cell or cell type. Among the main characteristics of proteins is that it allows a diverse set of functions such as the ability to bind other molecules specifically and tightly. The binding site in the region of the protein is responsible for binding another molecule. The binding site is also known as depression or pocket on the molecule surface. The tertiary structure of proteins influences their binding ability. The binding ability defines the pocket of the binding site and also the chemical properties of the surrounding amino acids' side chains.

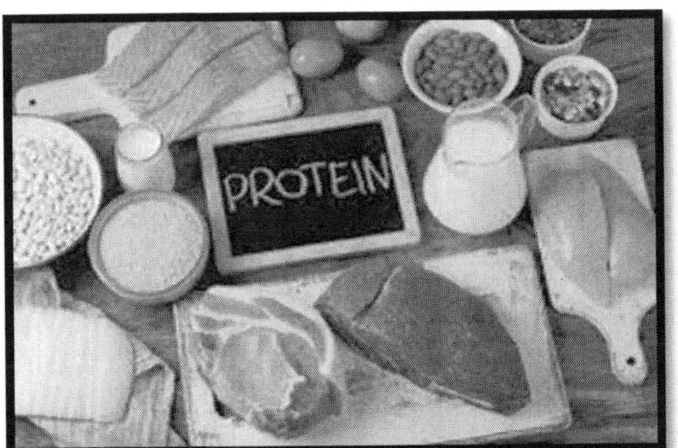

Figure 4.5: There are various sources of protein in the diet.

Protein binding is often described as extraordinarily tight and specific. This is demonstrated by ribonuclease inhibitor protein binds to human angiogenin with a sub-femtomolar dissociation constant. However, it does not bind at all to the amphibian homolog on conase. Any extreme minor chemical changes such as adding a single methyl group to a binding partner may at times suffice to nearly eliminate binding. Proteins possess the ability to bind to other proteins as well as other small-molecule substrates. In the case where proteins specifically bind to other copies of the same molecule, they can oligomerize resulting in the formation of fibrils. This is known to occur in structural proteins that consist of globular monomers that self-associate resulting in the formation of rigid fibers. Interactions between proteins are useful in regulating enzymatic activity, controlling the progression through the cell cycle, and allowing the assembly of large protein complexes that carry out several closely related reactions with a common biological function (Ballester-Sánchez *et al.*, 2019).

Binding can also extend to or integrate into cell membranes. The induction of conformational changes in proteins is affected by the ability of binding partners. This allows the construction of enormously complex signaling networks. It is important to note that interactions between proteins are reversible. They are heavily dependent on the availability of different groups of partner proteins to form aggregates with the ability to carry out discrete sets of functions. A study of the interactions between specific proteins is useful in understanding important aspects of cellular function and the properties that distinguish particular cell types.

4.9 ENZYMES

Proteins play an important role in the cell as enzymes. Enzymes are involved in the catalysis of chemical reactions. Among the characteristics of enzymes is that they are highly specific and accelerate one or a few chemical reactions. Enzymes are greatly involved in several reactions such as metabolism and manipulation of DNA in processes such as transcription, DNA repair, and DNA replication. Certain enzymes act on proteins to remove or add chemical groups through a process known as post-translational modification. Enzymes catalyze about 4,000 reactions. The rate of acceleration of reactions conferred by enzymatic catalysis is usually enormous with the yield going as high as a 1017-fold increase in rate over the uncatalyzed reaction. This is the case in orotate decarboxylase. A substrate is a name given to the molecule bound and acted upon by enzymes (Bacon & Hobson, 2014). Enzymes are known to have various kinds of amino acids. In the enzymes, a small fraction of the residues is known to come in contact with the substrate. An even smaller fraction of about three to four residues is directly involved in catalysis. The region in which the enzymes bind to the substrate and contain the catalytic residues are referred to as active sites. There are different members of the class of proteins. Among them is dirigent protein. Such kinds of proteins dictate the stereochemistry of a compound synthesized by other enzymes.

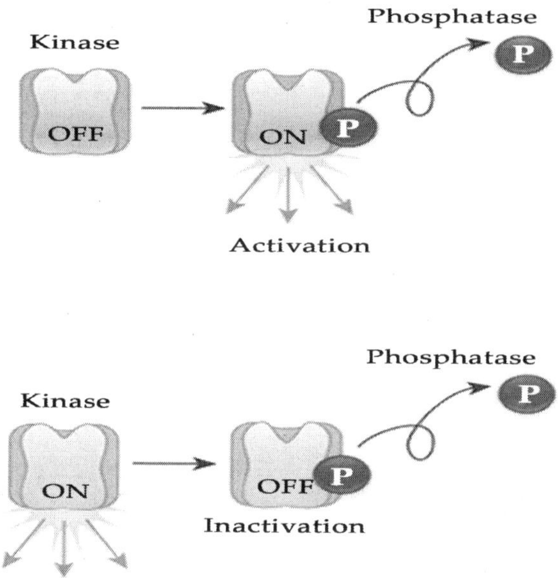

Figure 4.6: Enzymes used in reactions are made from proteins.

4.10 LIGAND BINDING AND CELL SIGNALING

There are different kinds of proteins involved in processes such as signal transduction and cell signaling. For proteins such as insulin, they are extracellular proteins involved in the transmission of signals from the cell where they were synthesized into other cells in distant tissues. There are membrane proteins that function as a receptor. The main role of such proteins is to bind a signaling molecule and also induce a biochemical response in the cell. In most cases, the receptors have a binding site exposed on the surface of cells and an effector domain within the cell. The effector domain may have enzymatic activity or may undergo a conformational change detected by other proteins within the cell.

Proteins are also utilized in the body in the form of antibodies. Antibodies are defined as protein components of an adaptive immune system whose main function is to bind antigens and foreign substances in the body. They can also target the antigens for destruction (Cassani et al., 2020). Antibodies are usually secreted into the extracellular environment and can also be anchored in the membranes of specialized B cells known as plasma cells. Antibodies are very different from enzymes in that enzymes are limited in their binding affinity for their substrates by the necessity of conducting their reaction which is not exhibited in antibodies. This means that the binding affinity of antibodies to their target is extraordinarily high.

There are several ligand transport proteins involved in the binding of particular small biomolecules. They transport them to other locations in the body of any multicellular organisms. Such proteins need to possess a high binding affinity in the presence of their ligand in high concentration. They should also release the ligand when present at low concentrations in the target tissue. A canonical example of a ligand-binding protein is hemoglobin. Hemoglobin is involved in the transportation of oxygen from the lungs to other organs and tissues in all vertebrates. They are said to be close to homologs in every biological kingdom. An example of sugar-binding proteins is a lectin. They are highly specific for their sugar moieties. Lectins play an important role in the biological recognition phenomenon that involves proteins and cells. Examples of highly specific binding proteins are hormones and receptors. Other proteins that could serve as ligand transport proteins are transmembrane. They can alter the permeability of the cell membrane to ions and small molecules (Bulaj *et al.,* 2016). The membrane on its own has a hydrophobic core through which charged or polar molecules cannot diffuse. Membrane proteins are also known to contain internal channels that allow the molecules to exit and enter the cell. The ion channel proteins are usually specialized to select for only a particular ion, for example, sodium and potassium channels often discriminate for only one of the two ions.

4.11 STRUCTURAL PROTEINS

Such kinds of proteins confer rigidity and stiffness to otherwise-fluid biological components. A large number of structural proteins are fibrous proteins. They include elastin and collagen. They are all critical components of connective tissue such as cartilage. Keratin is usually found in filamentous or hard structures such as nails and hair. Globular proteins may play structural functions. Examples of globular proteins include tubulin and actin. They are soluble as monomers. They can also polymerize to form long and stiff fibers that make up the cytoskeleton. This allows body cells to maintain their shape and size. Motor proteins may also play structural functions. They include dynein, kinesin, and myosin. They can generate mechanical forces. These proteins are useful in the cellular motility of single-celled organisms and also the sperm of multicellular organisms that reproduce sexually. These proteins can generate forces that can be exerted through the contraction of muscles. They play essential roles in intracellular transport.

Among the other uses of proteins include their use in growth and maintenance. Our body tissues need proteins to facilitate growth and maintenance. Usually, the body's proteins are in a constant state of turnover. Normally, the body breaks down the same amount of proteins that are used in building and repairing tissues. However, there are cases where the body breaks down large amounts of proteins which can create increasing the amount needed by the body. This mostly occurs during periods of illness, when breastfeeding, and during pregnancy. Large amounts of proteins are needed by people recovering from an injury or surgery, athletes, and older adults.

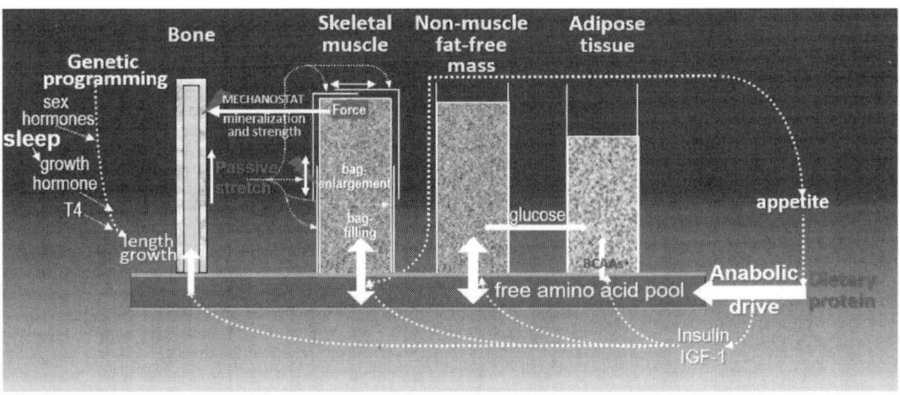

Figure 4.7: Proteins facilitate growth and repair in the body.

(Source: Millward DJ., 2021)

Proteins are used to facilitate biochemical reactions. This mostly involves enzymes. They are a group of proteins that aid the thousands of biochemical reactions that take place in and out of body cells. Enzymes have been structured such that they can combine with other molecules inside the cell also known as substrates. Enzymes catalyze reactions that are very important to metabolism. Enzymes can also function outside of their cells. They include digestive enzymes such as sucrase and lactase all of which are used in digesting sugar. Some enzymes need other molecules such as minerals or vitamins for a reaction to take place. Some of the bodily functions that are dependent on enzymes include digestion, blood clotting, muscle contraction, and energy production. When these enzymes are not well utilized, the person may suffer from diseases (Bis-Souza *et al.,* 2019).

Proteins can also act as a messenger. As mentioned earlier, some hormones are protein in nature. Hormones are chemical messengers that aid the communication between body organs, tissues, and cells. Hormones are made and secreted by endocrine glands or tissues. They are then transported in the blood to target organs and tissues where they bind to protein receptors on the cell surface. Hormones can be placed into three main groups namely amines, steroids, and peptides and protein. Amines are made from individual amino acids or tyrosine. This is used to help make hormones related to metabolism and sleep. Steroids are hormones made from fat cholesterol. Examples of hormones that are steroid-based include estrogen, testosterone, and sex hormones. Peptides and proteins are hormones made from chains of amino acids. They usually range from a few to several hundred. A large percentage of the body's hormones are protein and polypeptide-based.

Some examples of hormones include insulin which is involved in signaling the uptake of glucose and sugar into the cell, ACTH which is involved in the stimulation of the release of cortisol and a key factor in metabolism, and ADH which signals the kidneys to reabsorb water, hGH is a hormone that stimulates the growth of various tissues such as bone and glucagon which is a hormone that signals the breakdown of stored glucose in the liver.

Proteins are useful in providing structure. There are proteins known to be fibrous and provide both tissues and cells with stiffness and rigidity. Some of these proteins include elastin, collagen, and keratin. They are known to be useful in forming the connective framework for certain structures in the body. Among the major structural proteins is keratin found in nails, hair, and skin. Collagen is also among the most important proteins in the body (Bis-Souza *et al.*, 2019). It is the structural protein in skin, ligaments, tendons, and bones. When collagen is compared to elastin, is found to be less flexible. Elastin is known to have high elasticity that allows many tissues in the body to return to the original shape after they experience stretching or contracting. This is the case in the uterus, arteries, and lungs.

Index (GI) is a measurement of how rapidly sugar enters the bloodstream. The glycemic response is characterized by a significant increase in blood sugar after carbohydrate consumption.

A meal's glycemic index indicates how much postprandial glucose levels rise. Highly refined carbohydrates cause a more rapid and widespread rise in blood sugar than whole grains that have not been highly refined. Increased plasma insulin levels are linked to higher glycemic reactions, which are thought to contribute to metabolic syndrome and infertility.

Diets with a high glycemic index or a high glycemic load appear to increase the risk of type 2 diabetes and coronary artery disease, especially in insulin-resistant women (Fabani *et al*., 2013). Milling removes a significant amount of fiber and minerals, potentially contributing to the negative effects of highly processed grains.

Whole grains, whole grain meals, fruits, vegetables, and legumes, on the other hand, are high in fiber, vitamins, minerals, and phytonutrients, as well as complex carbs that take longer to digest. Whole grains and high-fiber cereals are less likely than highly processed grains to cause cardiovascular disease and type 2 diabetes. While it is difficult to prove that a high-fiber diet reduces the risk of colon cancer, it has been linked to less constipation and diverticular disease.

5.4 PROTEIN

Amino acids are fed to metabolic systems that are involved in protein synthesis and repair, regardless of whether they are derived from animal or plant protein. Protein, on the other hand, is rarely consumed in its natural condition. Rather, it has been fortified with a variety of vitamins and minerals. The quantity and quality of lipids, carbohydrates, salt, and other nutrients in the "protein package" may have a long-term impact on health. According to the Nurses' Health Study, increasing protein intake from beans, nuts, seeds, and other sources while avoiding easily digested carbohydrates lowers the risk of heart disease (Lin *et al*., 2010). According to that study, increasing animal protein consumption while decreasing carbohydrate consumption did not reduce the risk of heart disease due to the lipids and other nutrients included in animal protein.

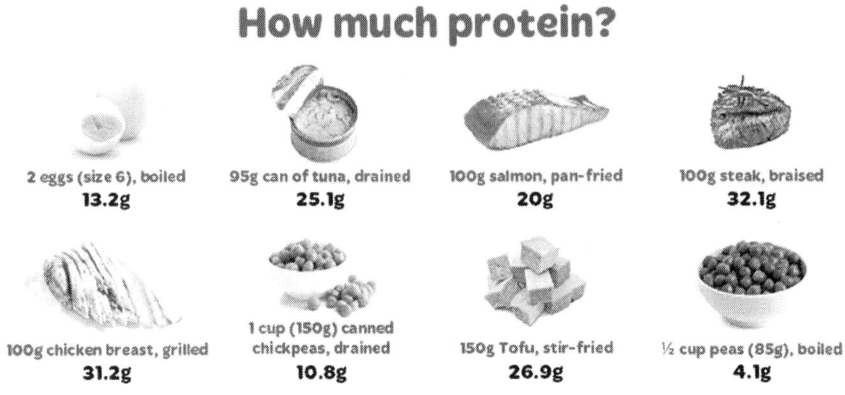

Figure 5.3: Protein.

5.5 FRUITS AND VEGETABLES

"Eat more fruits and vegetables," as the adage goes. This is fantastic advice that is supported by a large body of data. Fruits and vegetables provide fiber, slowly digested carbohydrates, vitamins and minerals, and phytonutrients that have been linked to a lower risk of cardiovascular disease, vision loss from cataracts and macular degeneration, and bowel function maintenance. Consumption of fruits and vegetables has been linked to a decreased risk of cancer. While fruits and vegetables may not have a broad anticancer effect, they may aid in the treatment of certain cancers such as esophageal, stomach, lung, and colorectal cancer (Linares *et al.*, 2017). Consume a diverse range of fruits and vegetables, with at least five servings per day, recommended—the more, the merrier. One out of every four people in the United States is affected by this disease.

5.6 BEVERAGES

It is preferable to drink a beverage that is low in calories and additives. Water meets all of these requirements. It costs less than a cent per glass when purchased directly from the tap. Tea and coffee are the most popular beverages after water. Both are extremely safe and have been linked to a lower risk of type 2 diabetes, kidney stones, gallstones, cardiovascular disease, and some cancers. Both alcoholic and sugar-sweetened beverages are hazardous. A 12-ounce can of sugar-sweetened cola contains eight to ten teaspoons of sugar or 120–150 "empty" calories. Sugary beverages have been linked to obesity, type 2 diabetes, heart disease, and gout. Moderate alcohol consumption has been linked to a lower risk of heart disease and type 2 diabetes. Moderate alcohol use, on the other hand, has been associated with an increased risk of breast cancer (López *et al.*, 2019). A high-folate diet, on the other hand, may help to reduce this risk. According to the Nurses' Health Study, women with a total folate intake of less than 300 g/d had the highest risk of breast cancer, compared to 15 g/d, the amount of alcohol in one "typical" drink. For multivariate relative risk, the 95 percent confidence interval is 1.15–1.50.

5.7 VITAMINS AND ELEMENTS

A well-balanced diet contains all of the vitamins, minerals, and other micronutrients needed for good health. However, many women in the United States are malnourished, with a disproportionate share of impoverished women among them. As a consequence, the majority of women may prevent nutritional shortfalls by taking a multivitamin-multimineral supplement consistently.

Iron supplements, which are frequently included in these formulations, are required by premenopausal women, who account for between 9 and 11 percent of the population. The likelihood of neural tube defects is lowered by roughly 70 percent when supplemental folic acid is provided during pregnancy. All women of reproductive age should take folic acid supplements containing 400 to 800 micrograms of folic acid per day, or 4 milligrams if your baby has a neural tube problem, according to current recommendations (Karioti *et al.,* 2015).

Calcium levels in the body affect bone strength. The actual quantity of calcium needed by an individual is debatable. 400 mg per day is prescribed by the World Health Organization. Women over the age of 19 in the United Kingdom are urged to take 700 mg of vitamin D daily. Adult women in the United States should take 1,500 mg of calcium per day, the bulk of which should come from low-fat or fat-free dairy products. Calcium supplements are calorie and fat-free sources of calcium.

Exercise and vitamin D, for example, are equally as necessary for bone health as calcium. There is emerging evidence that current vitamin D levels are insufficient and that taking 1,000 international units of vitamin D per day can help prevent fractures, heart disease, and cancer. Excessive vitamin A consumption has been connected to an increased risk of hip fracture, most likely as a result of vitamin D competition. Consuming substantially more than the current Dietary Reference Intake of 700 g per day, on the other hand, is associated with larger risk. Given this issue, it is advised that you take a multivitamin with a high dose of vitamin A in the form of beta-carotene.

5.8 WEIGHT CONTROL AND EXERCISE

A web of health and disease is woven into the web of body weight. Obesity has been linked to an increased risk of developing several chronic diseases. A BMI of 25 kg/m2 or higher increases the risk of hypertension and cardiovascular disease, diabetes, various cancers, gallstones, sleep apnea, pregnancy complications, infertility, and premature death. A BMI of 18–25 kg/m2 is currently recommended by national standards, and optimal health is achieved by limiting weight gain during maturation. Calorie intake and expenditure have a direct impact on a person's ability to maintain or lose weight healthily. Controlling portion size is essential for weight loss (Francesconi, 2007). It is possible to lose weight by consuming fewer sugary beverages and Tran's fats and increasing your intake of dietary fiber. Regular exercise and avoiding excessive lethargy, such as excessive television viewing, are also important weight-control strategies. A welcoming social and physical environment is also required.

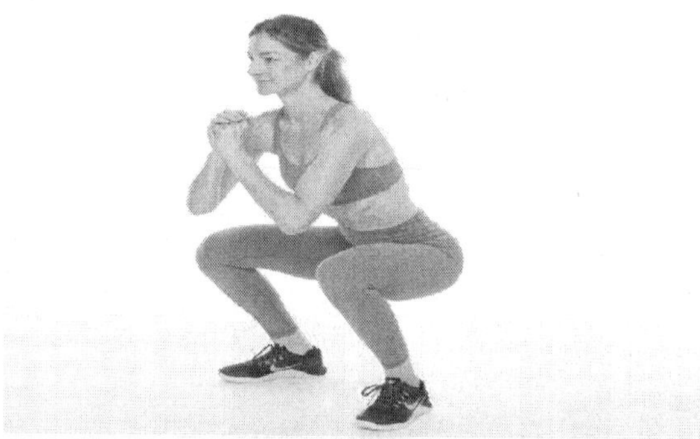

Figure 5.4: Exercise.

5.9 PATTERNS OF DIET

While research on lipids, carbs, and certain vitamins and minerals has been valuable, it has also led to countless dead ends and considerable

Ensuring you're eating adequate protein will help you feel satiated for longer, which can be good for decreasing your calorie consumption, to begin with. Due to the straining process, Greek yogurt is lower in carbohydrates and lactose than plain yogurt. This makes it acceptable for folks who are lactose intolerant or on a low-carb diet.

Greek yogurt may be swapped for some of your favorite snacks or yogurt variations to obtain a healthy dose of protein and minerals. Ensure that the unflavored, basic types are chosen. Additional sugar and other less nutritional components may be present in flavored yogurt. If you don't have a list, don't go shopping (Francesconi, 2007). There are two major ways to go food shopping: Make a list of what you need to buy ahead of time so you don't arrive at the shop hungry. Hunger can lead to spontaneous purchases, and it can also lead to the purchase of even more poor-quality food products. It's consequently crucial that you write down everything you'll need in advance. You'll not only save money, but you'll also buy nutritious food for your household if you follow your plan and adhere to it. It's recommended to have eggs for breakfast every day.

Having eggs for breakfast is a terrific idea because they can be utilized for several things.

The protein of the highest quality and other vital elements, such as choline, are abundant in these meals. When comparing several calorie-matched meals, eggs come out on top when looking at the data. Eggs in the morning make you feel more fulfilled. As a result, consumers have been proven to consume fewer calories following meals as a result of this. If you're seeking to lose weight, it might be highly beneficial. It was shown that having an egg-based breakfast lowered hunger signals and reduced the number of calories ingested later in the day than eating cereal for lunch. Because of this, a simple adjustment to eggs for your morning meal can have a huge influence on your health.

Add additional protein to your diet: Protein is usually considered the most important nutrient, and there is some evidence to support this. It's typically called the most gratifying macronutrient because of its capacity to alter your appetite and fullness hormones. People with obesity who ate a high-protein, low-carb dinner had lower levels of ghrelin, the hunger hormone, than those who ate a high-carb meal.

Protein, on the other hand, helps you retain muscle mass and may also help you burn a few extra calories each day. It's also crucial if you want to avoid muscle loss that occurs with losing weight and becoming older

(Linares *et al.*, 2017).If you want to reduce weight, make an effort to include a protein source in each meal and snack you eat. You'll have fewer cravings, feel fuller for longer, and be less inclined to overeat as a consequence of this method.

- Milk products, almonds, and peanut butter are all healthy sources of protein; eggs, lentils, and lean meat are other acceptable possibilities.
- Keep yourself hydrated!
- Drinking sufficient water is vital to your general well-being.
- Many studies have shown that drinking water can help you lose weight and keep it off, and it may even help you burn a few additional calories each day.
- Drinking water before a meal has also been demonstrated to lessen the quantity of food you eat during the subsequent meal.
- The most essential thing to remember is to drink water rather than other beverages. This might have a substantial influence on your sugar and calorie consumption.
- Drinking water daily may also enhance the quality of your meals and help you eat fewer calories from drinks.
- As an alternative to grilling or frying, consider baking or roasting your dish instead
- The manner you cook your meals might have a big influence on your health.
- Cooking meat and fish on the grill, broiling, frying, or deep-frying is a time-honored practice.
- Several substances can be toxic when used in cooking, though (López et al., 2019). Among them are polycyclic aromatic hydrocarbons, end products of advanced glycation, and heterocyclic amines, to mention a few.

Several of these drugs have been related to cancer and heart disease, among other major health consequences.

- Baking, broiling, poaching, pressure cooking, simmering, slow cooking, stewing, and sous-vide are some of the healthier cooking techniques.
- As a consequence, the development of these hazardous compounds is delayed and your meals may become healthier as a result.

- The odd grilled or deep-fried item is great, but it's better to utilize these methods infrequently.
- Supplement your diet with vitamin D and omega-3 fatty acids (Karioti et al., 2015).
- An estimated 1 billion individuals throughout the world suffer from vitamin D insufficiency.
- Because of its significance in bone health and immune system function, fat-soluble vitamin D is a need. Vitamin D can be present in every cell of your body, demonstrating its use.
- Only a few meals are required to acquire the recommended quantity of vitamin D, and the greatest source is fatty fish.
- This is another prevalent shortage, in addition to the omega-3 fatty acids present in fatty fish. Some of the activities they play in the body include reducing inflammation, improving heart health, and maintaining healthy brain function.
- In the Western diet, omega-6 fatty acids, which produce inflammation, have been related to a range of chronic disorders. You may utilize omega-3 fatty acids to assist reduce inflammation and maintaining a more balanced condition in your body.
- If you don't consume fish daily and are concerned about your health, you may need to take a supplement. Supplements containing both omega-3 fatty acids and vitamin D3 are widely available.
- Replace your favorite fast food restaurant with this one.
- When you dine out, you don't have to consume bad food.
- Instead of your normal fast-food restaurant, consider heading to a healthier option.
- A variety of healthy fast-food restaurants and fusion kitchens provide healthful and appetizing meals. They may be found all over the place (Khorram & Ramezanian, 2021).
- They could be a good option for your favorite burger or pizza establishment. Furthermore, these meals are typically reasonably priced.
- At the absolute least, one new healthy recipe should be tried once a week.

- When faced with the difficulty of deciding what to eat for supper, many individuals choose to eat the same foods again and over. If you're like most people, you've been preparing the same meals without even thinking about it.
- Even if it's a bad dinner, trying something new may be a fun way to spice up your diet.
- Make an effort at least once a week to attempt a new healthful recipe. Change your eating habits to incorporate new and healthier meals into your everyday routine (Haque et al., 2020).
- Fresh ingredients, herbs, and spices, on the other hand, maybe utilized to make a healthier version of a popular dish, and French fries are preferred to boiled potatoes.
- Potatoes are commonly offered as a side dish with other significant dishes in many cultures. The technique of cooking, on the other hand, has a substantial influence on the health repercussions of these meals.
- Baked potatoes have 93 calories per 3.5 ounces (100 grams), but French fries have more than three times that amount.
- Deep-fried French fries include aldehydes and Trans fats as well.
- You may use roasted or boiled potatoes for French fries to conserve calories and eliminate possibly dangerous additives.
- Begin by eating a range of brightly colored fruits and vegetables.
- Serving your greens as the first dish is a terrific method to guarantee that you consume them.
- Eating your greens while hungry is a certain way to devour them all. As a result of this shift in habit, you may wind up eating fewer of the meal's other, possibly dangerous, components (Hou & Xu, 2022).
- It may result in a decrease in your overall calorie intake, which may result in weight loss.
- Furthermore, studies have shown that eating veggies before a high-carbohydrate meal raises blood sugar levels.

CHAPTER 5

PRACTICAL ADVICE ON MAINTAINING A HEALTHY DIET

CONTENTS

5.1 INTRODUCTION

A healthy diet can help people avoid malnutrition as well as a variety of food-related diseases and disorders throughout their lives. The rise of refined and high-energy meals, as well as processed foods, has, nevertheless, resulted in a variety of lifestyle modifications. Diabetes, cardiovascular disease, and cancer are all diet-related diseases that can be avoided by eating well (Pop *et al*., 2019). Furthermore, reducing calorie intake and avoiding processed foods and Trans fats, may help people reduce their risk of developing these diseases. Patients frequently inquire, "How do I know if I'm eating a healthy diet?"

As a result of an avalanche of data and inconsistent findings across studies, many physicians may struggle to find a solution to this simple but difficult problem. In diet literature and the media, there are a lot of misconceptions regarding healthy eating. That is unfortunate because there are now enough reliable data points to develop simple but persuasive dietary recommendations. The average woman in the United States and other developed countries can expect to live for 80 years or more. Consuming the calories required to survive, develop, and repair the body is insufficient at this stage of life. Chronic diseases such as heart disease, cancer, osteoporosis, and aging-related vision loss can all be influenced by the foods that provide these calories.

While much is still unknown about the role of specific nutrients in lowering the risk of chronic disease, growing evidence suggests that eating whole grains, legumes, vegetables, and fruits while avoiding red meat, full-fat dairy products, and sugary foods and beverages is beneficial. These diets have been linked to a lower risk of developing several chronic illnesses. Of course, diet is only one way to prevent disease. Calorie restrictions to maintain a healthy weight, regular physical activity, and quitting smoking are all important measures (Odhaib et al., 2021). Women who followed a healthy lifestyle pattern that included these four approaches were 80 percent less likely than all other women in the study to develop cardiovascular diseases over 14 years, according to Nurses' Health Research.

According to a separate study, the Health Professionals Follow-up Study, men benefited from similar healthy choices, even if they were taking blood pressure or cholesterol-lowering medications. This page examines evidence-based eating patterns and nutritional components. In addition, we investigate the association between nutrition and fertility, pregnancy, and weight reduction in three different contexts.

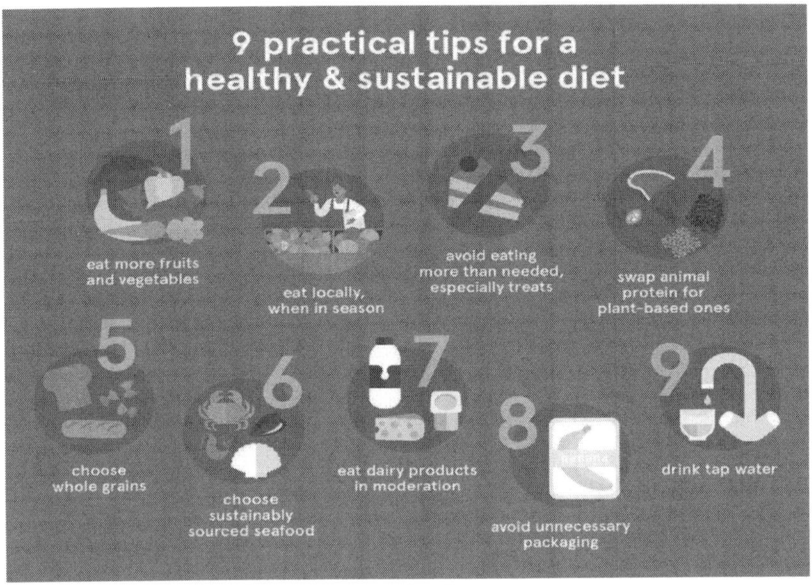

Figure 5.1: 9 practical tips for a healthy and sustainable diet.

5.2 THE DIET INCLUDES FAT

Dietary fat is a nutrient that is often misunderstood and overlooked. There have been misconceptions and messages that "fat is bad" since the 1960s. As a result of this possibly harmful oversimplification, thousands of fat-free yet calorie-dense meals, as well as hundreds of totally worthless diets, have been devised. It has also contributed to the obesity and type 2 diabetes epidemics. The idea that "fat is deleterious" is erroneous as there are four unique forms of dietary fat, each having a different influence on health. Tran's fats are detrimental to your heart and general wellness. They are made with partially hydrogenated oils (Murdoch *et al.,* 2000). These lipids, which are primarily produced, enhance dangerous low-density lipoprotein cholesterol while reducing good high-density lipoprotein cholesterol, promote inflammation, and induce a range of other changes that damage arteries and have an influence on cardiovascular health. Tran's fat intake has been associated with cardiovascular disease, type 2 diabetes, gallstones, dementia, and weight gain. Saturated fats, common in red meat and dairy products, enhance LDL cholesterol and lowering HDL. Consumption of low-saturated fat is consistent with a healthy diet, whereas consumption of high-saturated fat has been associated with cardiovascular disease.

Monounsaturated and polyunsaturated fats, especially polyunsaturated omega-3 fatty acids found in vegetable oils, seeds, nuts, whole grains, and seafood, are vital components of a balanced diet that aid promote heart health. Polyunsaturated fats, as opposed to saturated and trans fats, can help decrease bad LDL cholesterol while boosting good HDL, enhancing insulin sensitivity, and regulating cardiac rhythms. No evidence eating fat increases the likelihood of having a chronic illness. Polyunsaturated and monounsaturated fat diets have been demonstrated to be particularly favorable when low in Trans and saturated fats and rich in polyunsaturated and monounsaturated fats (Multari *et al.,* 2015). While there is no definite evidence on the appropriate fat proportions in the diet, it has been shown that a diet low in trans and saturated fats and rich in unsaturated fats lessens the risk of heart disease and diabetes.

5.3 CARBOHYDRATES

While dietary fat consumption in the United States has decreased from 45% in 1965 to around 34% today, carbohydrate consumption has increased. The majority of the extra carbohydrates came from highly processed cereals. White flour and white rice are nutritionally inferior to whole grains because they lack fiber, healthy fats, and a variety of vitamins, minerals, and phytonutrients. A high-processed-grain diet has been associated with higher triglyceride levels and lower HDL cholesterol levels.

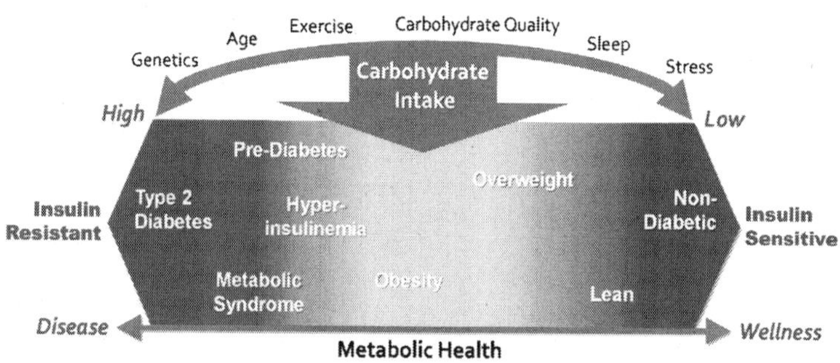

Figure 5.2: Carbohydrates.

(Source: Volek JS, Phinney SD., et, al.,2021)

Insulin resistance, which is common during pregnancy, may aggravate these negative effects. Insulin resistance and type 2 diabetes are becoming more common in the United States and across the world. The Glycemic

Proteins help the body maintain proper pH. Proteins are very essential in regulating the concentrations of bases and acids in the blood and other body fluids. A pH scale is used in measuring the balance between bases and acids. The scale ranges from 0 to 14 with the acidic being 0-7 and 7-14 being the alkaline. Substances in the body have different pH levels. For instance, tomato juice has a pH of 4, black coffee is at 5, human blood is at 7.4, milk of magnesia at 10, and soapy water at 12. There are different kinds of buffeting systems that allows bodily fluids to maintain normal pH ranges. This is done because a constant pH is very essential. Any slight changes in pH could be harmful or potentially deadly. One method of pH regulation is with proteins. Hemoglobin is a protein that makes up red blood cells. It is known to bind small amounts of acid thereby helping maintain the normal pH value of blood. Other buffer systems in the body include bicarbonate and phosphate.

Proteins are useful in balancing body fluids. They can regulate body processes to maintain fluid balance. Some of the proteins in the blood that help maintain the body's fluid balance are globulin and albumin. They maintain the balance by retaining and attracting water. There is a decrease in the levels of albumin and globulin when insufficient amounts of protein are consumed (Yousuf *et al.*, 2021). As a result, such proteins can no longer keep blood in blood vessels and the fluid is forced into spaces between cells. A buildup of fluid in between the spaces in the cells causes edema or swelling more so in the stomach region. This is considered a form of severe protein malnutrition called kwashiorkor. Kwashiorkor is a disease that develops when an individual consumes enough calories but does not consume sufficient amounts of proteins. This kind of disease is rare in developed regions of the world. It is often noted in areas of starvation.

Proteins are useful in boosting immune health. There are actively involved in the formation of antibodies and immunoglobulins useful in fighting infections. Antibodies are special proteins found in the blood that help protect the body from harmful invaders such as viruses and bacteria. In the case where foreign invaders are entering the cells, the body produces antibodies that tag them for elimination. In the absence of such antibodies, viruses and bacteria would be free to multiply and overwhelm the body leading to diseases. When the body produces antibodies against a given virus or bacteria, the cells will never forget how to make them. This enables the antibodies to respond quickly in light of a disease agent invasion in the body. As a result, the body develops immunity against diseases they are exposed to.

Proteins are involved in the transportation and storage of nutrients. Proteins involved in the transportation of proteins carry substances throughout the bloodstream such as into the cells, out of cells, or within the bed. Among the substances transported by proteins include nutrients such as minerals or vitamins, oxygen, cholesterol, and blood sugar. A good example is when hemoglobin which is a protein involved in the transportation of oxygen from the lungs to body tissues. Protein glucose transporters are used in moving glucose to body cells while lipoproteins transport fats and cholesterol in the blood (Walker *et al.,* 2015). By nature, protein transporters are specific. This means that they will bind to a specific substrate. This means that a proton transporter that moves cholesterol will not move glucose. Other than transportation, proteins also have storage roles. Ferritin is an example of a storage protein that stores ions. Another protein that plays the same role is casein. It is considered a principal protein in milk that facilitates growth in babies.

Proteins can also be considered a source of energy. They can be able to supply a sufficient amount of energy. They are known to contain four calories per gram. This is the same amount of energy provided by carbohydrates. A large amount of energy in the body is supplied by fats usually nine calories per gram. However, it is not convenient for the body to use proteins as a source of energy as it is a valuable nutrient that is widely used throughout the body. For this reason, both fats and carbs are considered to be better sources of energy as the body can maintain the reserves for use as fuel. They are also metabolized more efficiently compared to proteins. However, it is important to note that proteins can supply the body with very little of the energy needed in normal circumstances. During fasting, the body breaks down the skeleton muscle. This allows the amino acids to supply the body with energy. Our bodies can use amino acids from broken-down skeletal muscle when there are low amounts of carbohydrates in the body. This mostly occurs after exhaustive exercise or when an individual does not consume sufficient amounts of calories in general.

4.12 UTILIZATION OF FRUITS AND VEGETABLES

Among the important elements to be incorporated into the diet are fruits and vegetables. By nature, fruits and vegetables contain minerals and vitamins useful in keeping people healthy. They are also useful in protecting the body from diseases. People can benefit from eating more vegetables and fruits as part of a well-balanced, regular diet and healthy active lifestyle. There are different kinds of vegetables and fruits and there are different ways to prepare, cook and serve them. It is required vat an average person consumes at least five servings of vegetables and two serves of fruit each day. There are different colors and varieties of fruits.

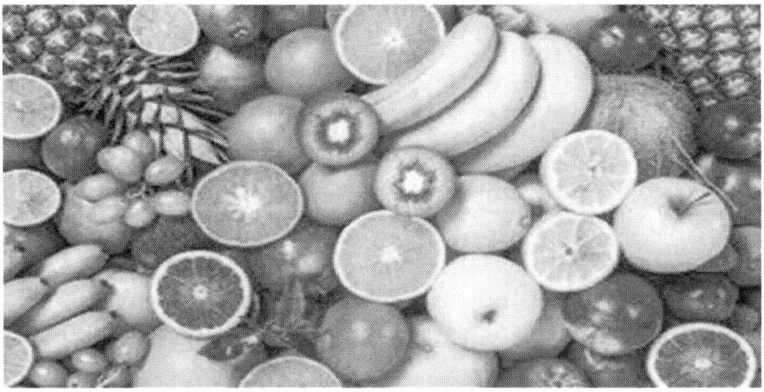

Figure 4.8: There are various nutrients and minerals in the body.

A single serving of vegetables is about a cup of raw salad vegetables or half a cup of cooked ones. A medium piece of fruit is a serving of fruit. There are different kinds of vitamins and minerals in vegetables and fruits. They are all good for our health. Examples of vitamins include vitamin A, vitamin C, and Vitamin E, folic acid, phosphorus, zinc, and magnesium. Folic acid is useful in reducing blood levels of homocysteine which is a substance that is a risk factor for coronary heart disease. The vitamins and minerals found in vegetables and fruits are useful in protecting the body from some types of cancers, reducing risks of digestive and eye problems, and reducing risks of stroke and heart disease. They are known to have a positive effect on blood sugar as it helps keeps our appetite in check (Vanbergen & Initiative, 2013). Consumption of non-starchy vegetables and fruits such as green leafy vegetables, pears, and apples may lead to weight loss. They are known to have low glycemic loads useful in preventing blood sugar spikes that can increase hunger. There are at least nine different families of vegetables and fruits in existence. They all have potentially hundreds of different plant compounds known to be beneficial to human health. For this reason, an individual is advised to eat different fruits of different colors and types so that the body can get the mix of nutrients it needs. This ensures the body gets diversity of beneficial plant chemicals and also creates eye-appealing meals.

The utilization of fruits and vegetables is for treating and preventing diseases. Among the diseases that can be prevented through the consumption of fruits and vegetables is cardiovascular disease. There is sufficient evidence to prove that diet rich in vegetables and fruits can lower the risks of stroke and heart disease. There were cohort studies involving 469,551 participants that saw that consumption of large amounts of vegetables and fruits is associated with reduced risks of death from cardiovascular disease. The average reduction of risk is 4% for each additional serving per day of vegetables and fruits. Currently, the longest and largest study was done as part of the Harvard-based Nurses' Health Study and Health Professional Follow-up Study which involved about 110,000 women and men whose health and dietary habits were followed for 14 years.

There are reduced chances of development of cardiovascular disease when the average daily intake of fruits and vegetables is high. When those in the lowest category of fruit and vegetable intake are compared to those on the higher side, those who averaged 8 or more servings in a day were found to be 30% less likely to have a stroke or heart attack. Fruits and vegetables are known to contribute to this. However, green leafy vegetables such as mustard greens, Swiss chard, spinach, and lettuce are strongly associated with decreased risk of cardiovascular disease. Kale, bok choy, Brussels sprouts, cabbage, cauliflower, and broccoli are collectively known as cruciferous vegetables, and citrus fruits such as grapefruits, lines, lemons, and oranges have made important contributions (Turner & Thompson, 2013). The results from studies done at Harvard and other long-term studies in Europe and U.S were combined. More emphasis was placed on coronary heart disease and stroke separately and fruits and vegetables were found to have similar protective effects. It was noted that individuals who ate more than 5 servings of fruits and vegetables per day had a 20% reduced risk of coronary heart disease and stroke when compared to those who are less than 3 servings per day.

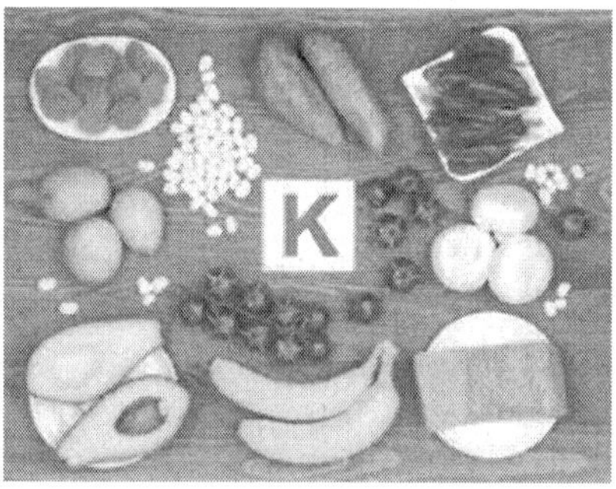

Figure 4.9: Fruits and vegetables can be used to reduce high blood pressure.

misunderstanding about what constitutes a healthy diet. People eat food rather than nutrition, according to one of the most frequent theories. Individuals' eating habits are also pretty consistent. While analyzing dietary patterns is more challenging than studying nutrients, current research shows that some dietary patterns are favorable to long-term health. The traditional Western diet, which is heavy in red meat, highly processed grains, and sugar and low in fruits, vegetables, whole grains, and fiber, is one dietary pattern that is hazardous to long-term health (Khorram & Ramezanian, 2021). Numerous studies have proven a relationship between this eating pattern and atherosclerosis and several cardiovascular disorders, including heart attacks and strokes, peripheral vascular disease, and heart failure.

The DGA (Dietary Guidelines for Americans) gives precise suggestions. The regulations are modified every five years by a committee designated by the US Department of Agriculture. The procedure was administered by the Department of Health and Human Services. According to the USDA, the guidelines "give reliable information to persons two years of age and older about how good eating practices can enhance health and lower the chance of acquiring major chronic illnesses." The Food Guide Pyramid was established to make the rules more accessible to a larger audience. Unfortunately, this omnipresent billboard mirrored both American agriculture aims and nutritional beliefs. The Food Guide Pyramid abolished carbohydrates in favor of classifying red meat, poultry, fish, and legumes and instructing us to evaluate them based on total fat content. The Food Guide Pyramid, which did not discriminate between different forms of fat and instead urged customers to consume fat "in moderation," advised people to drink three glasses of low-fat milk or eat three pieces of various dairy products each day.

The Food Guide Pyramid was superseded in 2005 by the abstract MyPyramid, which can only be comprehended when paired with the associated Web site. The food industry hailed the abolition of food categories in favor of vertical stripes since the previous Food Guide Pyramid defined meals at the bottom as "good" and those at the top as "poor." The pattern suggests that all meals are nutritionally comparable from left to right. The Healthy Eating Pyramid, devised by nutrition specialists at Harvard School of Public Health using the most recent evidence, represents a healthy eating pattern. People who want to follow a pre-determined dietary pattern rather than designing their own utilizing the Healthy Eating Pyramid may benefit from a Mediterranean-style or DASH diet (Kadam & Prabhasankar, 2010).

5.9.1 Guidelines for the Mediterranean Diet

A traditional Mediterranean diet has been linked to a lower prevalence of heart disease and other chronic illnesses in countries bordering the Mediterranean Sea. Such diets are also responsive to shifting environmental circumstances. Those whose diets most closely resembled a traditional Mediterranean diet had lower risks of all-cause mortality, cardiovascular mortality, and cancer mortality than those who followed a Western diet, according to the 166,012 women who participated in the National Institutes of Health's AARP Diet and Health Study. Men went to a similar course. Smokers experienced a significantly greater impact. Furthermore, the Mediterranean diet has been shown to lower the risk of cancer, Parkinson's disease, and Alzheimer's disease. Furthermore, it has been linked to the treatment of asthma and rheumatoid arthritis symptoms. While there is no such thing as "the" Mediterranean diet, people who follow it should consume a lot of extra virgin olive oil, whole grains, fiber, fruits, vegetables, legumes, and nuts (Jacob *et al.,* 2020). Consumption includes small amounts of cheese and yogurt regularly; fish in varying proportions; and red meat, poultry, eggs, and sweets in moderation. Moderate amounts of red wine with meals are advised, as is regular physical activity.

In the 1990s, the National Heart, Lung, and Blood Institute launched DASHs (Dietary Approaches to Stop Hypertension), a randomized, controlled trial to see if specific dietary changes could help lower blood pressure. The DASH diet emphasizes fruits and vegetables as well as low-fat dairy products while limiting red meat, saturated fats, and sugar. The DASH diet reduced participants' systolic and diastolic blood pressures by 5.5 and 3 mm Hg, respectively, when compared to a traditional American diet. A low-sodium DASH diet was found to be significantly more effective, with results comparable to antihypertensive medication. Aside from decreasing blood pressure, the DASH diet has numerous other advantages. It was later established that it aids in weight reduction, decreases the risk of heart disease and stroke, and helps patients avoid kidney stones. Other diets, in addition to the Mediterranean and DASH diets, are being researched. The results of the Optimal Macronutrient Intake Trial to Prevent Heart Disease has been released. It has been proven that substituting protein or unsaturated fat for specific carbohydrates in a balanced diet lowers blood pressure, improves cholesterol levels, and lowers the risk of cardiovascular disease (Ibrahim *et al.*, 2015). The portfolio dietary plan was developed by University of Toronto experts. This mostly vegetarian diet reduced cholesterol by including soluble fiber-rich foods like oats, barley, psyllium, okra, and eggplant, as well as soy protein, whole almonds, and margarine modified with plant sterols. This cholesterol-lowering food collection reduced average LDL cholesterol levels by 29% while not affecting HDL cholesterol levels.

5.10 PREGNANCY AND DIET

Over 2 million American women experience infertility each year. Others are impoverished, while others comprehend the benefits of assisted reproductive technology. While farmers and ranchers have long recognized a link between diet and fertility in farm animals, little investigation has been undertaken on the human equivalent. The Nurses' Health Investigation has ended, the world's largest, longest, and most thorough diet and fertility investigation. The diet and fertility sub-study involved 18,555 women who reported a desire to start a family on a bimonthly Nurses' Health Study questionnaire; none of the women had previously experienced infertility. Over eight years, these women reported 25,217 pregnancies and/or pregnancy attempts ranging from a few weeks to more than twelve months. 3,209 women voiced concerns about infertility, with 438 being diagnosed with ovulatory infertility, the most frequent cause of female factor infertility. Eight dietary and lifestyle recommendations were related to a lower prevalence of ovulatory infertility in this nested case-control analysis.

The findings were revealed as part of a series of studies spanning several areas. Women in the top quintile of the "fertility diet" score had a significantly lower risk of ovulatory infertility and other causes of infertility than those in the lowest quintile. Combining five or more low-risk lifestyle factors, such as diet, weight management, and physical activity, was related to a 66 percent reduction in population-attributable risk and a 69 percent reduction in infertility owing to ovulatory disorders (Hou & Xu, 2022). A nutritious diet during pregnancy can boost the mother's health, lower the possibility of birth defects, promote normal fetal growth and development, and protect the growing child from chronic health difficulties. Women should follow the Dietary Guidelines for Americans both before and throughout pregnancy, according to the American College of Obstetrics and Gynecology and the American Dietetic Association.

Maintaining a healthy weight, increasing physical activity, supplementing with vitamins and minerals as needed, and refraining from alcohol, cigarettes, and other harmful substances are all crucial. Due to recent warnings about the risks of mercury in fish, some pregnant women have avoided shellfish.

Omega-3 fatty acids, which are abundant in a variety of fish species, however, have been demonstrated to stimulate embryonic development. Consumption of low-mercury fish in moderation during pregnancy has not been proven to generate difficulties. Pregnant and lactating women should consume no more than 12 ounces of mercury-free fish and shellfish per week, according to the Food and Drug Administration and the Environmental Protection Agency. Anchovies, catfish, flounder, mackerel, Pollock, salmon, sardines, shrimp, and tilapia are examples of low-mercury seafood.

Numerous more studies have underlined the important significance of omega-3 fatty acids and vitamin D in pregnancy. Jordan recommends pregnant women ingest 200–300 mg of DHA per day from safe dietary sources such as purified fish and algal oil supplements, as well as DHA-enhanced eggs for those who do not eat fish. Kendall-Tackett examines current research on omega-3 fatty acids and women's mental health, finding that EPA is effective in the treatment of depression and that EPA and DHA are safe for pregnant and postpartum women at low doses (Haque et al., 2020). Due to the hazards inherent with sun exposure, Kaludjerovic and Vieth's research reveals that low vitamin D intake during fetal development is hazardous to human health and gives current vitamin D supplementation recommendations.

5.11 CONTROL OF DIET AND WEIGHT

Almost any diet, at least initially, will result in weight loss if the dieter can consume fewer calories than she burns. Few dieters, on the other hand, can maintain a weight-loss regimen for an extended period. Because everyone's palates, dietary preferences, familial situations, and even inheritance differ, no single diet is suitable for everyone. A long-term dietary pattern that is good for the heart, bones, brain, intellect, and taste buds while also being good for the waistline is required. This diet should include a diverse range of meals with little restrictions or "special" products. According to evidence from randomized controlled trials, the nutritional content of a dietary pattern for weight reduction is far less important than the number of calories it provides. Participants in a head-to-head comparison of four diets loosely based on the Atkins, Ornish, and Mediterranean diets lost an average of 13.2 pounds and had a 2-inch reduction in waist circumference after six months, regardless of the plan. At 12 months, the majority of patients had begun to regain some of the weight they had lost. After two years, weight loss was comparable between those assigned to a 25% protein diet and those assigned to a 15% protein diet, as well as between those assigned to a 40% fat diet and those assigned to a 20% fat diet.

Within the intended range of 35 to 65 percent of calories from carbohydrates, carbohydrate consumption did not affect weight loss. Waist circumference changes were roughly identical across diet groups. Hunger, fullness, and meal pleasure were consistent across the board, as were cholesterol levels and other cardiovascular disease risk variables. It's critical to understand that these averages mask huge disparities in weight loss, with some patients losing 30 pounds or more while others gained weight during the experiment (Pop et al., 2019). This emphasizes the need of tailoring weight-loss therapy to the individual. Group treatment improved weight loss, indicating that behavioral, psychological, and social factors are more important than dietary balance in weight control.

5.12 DEVELOPMENTS IN FOOD CONSUMPTION

Significant food intake trends in the Netherlands, according to the Health Council and RIVM Reports. The documentary Our Food, Our Health examines how Dutch people have eaten over the years. The following is a list of these occurrences.

5.12.1 Changes in How People Consume Certain Foods

In 1997/98, the third National Food Consumption Survey was done to determine how much food the average individual consumes. Between 1987/88 and 1997/98, the following trends emerged: The average intake of staple foods such as bread, potatoes, vegetables, fruit, and meat dropped between 1987/88 and 1997/98. Vegetable consumption was shown to be the fastest declining. One-quarter of the Dutch population over the age of 12 ingested the recommended 150–200 grams of veggies per day in 1997/98. Non-bread cereals, milk and other dairy products, nuts and snacks, prepared meals, and non-alcoholic beverages all gained in popularity; but, prepared meals and non-alcoholic beverages remained especially popular. Fish consumption remained stable or grew slightly between 1987/88 and 1997/98. While one-quarter of the population eats fish at least once a week, the majority of the population does not do so regularly. According to the MORGEN Project, 10% of adult males interviewed in 1996 stated that they had never eaten fish, indicating a healthy long-term diet (Odhaib *et al.*, 2021). According to current sales projections, seafood consumption in the United States has lately climbed significantly.

5.12.2 Variations in the Number of Nutrients Eaten

According to the Netherlands' third National Food Consumption Survey, the typical Dutch diet between 1987/88 and 1997/98 had the following macronutrient composition and trend. A 4% reduction in average calorie consumption between 1987/88 and 1997/98 did not prevent an increase in the number of overweight or obese persons. Between 1987/88 and 1997/98, the Committee that developed this study found that this was the case because physical activity declined more than the energy level of the typical person's food intake. In both trials, Americans increased their fat consumption, as did the number of fatty acids in that fat. This fall in consumption was mostly due to a decrease in the quantity of mono-trans-unsaturated fats in hydrogenated vegetable oils.

Higher-fat products in the "oils, fats, and sauces," "milk," and "and poultry" categories appear to have been phased out in favor of lower-fat alternatives, which explains the less noticeable reduction in saturated fatty acid intake. Despite this, saturated fat accounted for more than 10% of total calories ingested by 95% of the population. Consumption of unsaturated fat by the average American was mainly consistent with the Dietary Reference Intakes Committee's guidelines. In the United States, dietary fatty acid consumption appears to be enough. On the other hand, precise data on -linoleic acid intake were insufficient. According to what is known about normal fish consumption, the average American diet has much fewer n-3 fatty acids than the required daily requirement (Murdoch *et al.,* 2000).

Only 17 percent of the population ingested enough fiber per megajoule of energy expenditure to fulfill the very minimal requirement of 3 grams of fiber per megajoule of energy expenditure. Fewer individuals consume bread, potatoes, fruits, and vegetables, making it more difficult for them to receive the necessary quantity of fiber.

Between 1987 and 1997, the nutritional density of the national diet dropped. Micronutrient consumption has fallen somewhat for the typical person. It is vital, however, to manage your folic acid consumption. Between 1990 and 1993, 60 percent of the adult population had inadequate folic acid status, if an acceptable blood homocysteine level was regarded as a measure of appropriate folic acid status. In this sense, we have been influenced by the fall in vegetable intake (Fabani *et al.*, 2013).

Between 1987/88 and 1997/98, iron intake decreased below the dietary reference value, notably among women of reproductive age. However, between 1990 and 1993, when these studies were undertaken, it was revealed that people with low or inadequate iron status were uncommon. We do not have any current data on salt consumption in the Netherlands that would allow us to establish the average intake in the nation. Between 1995 and 1997, sodium excretion measurements on 190 Dutch patients as part of the EPIC calibration experiment indicated an average daily sodium consumption of 3.9 grams. This equates to a daily salt consumption of around 9.8 grams.

5.13 NATIONAL FOOD CONSUMPTION SURVEY 2003

Young people's dietary habits were studied in 2003 as part of a larger study. Chapter 1 of the 2006 Dietary Guidelines for Americans Background Document summarizes the major findings of the survey. As previous food consumption surveys used a different methodology and style, the results from the 2003 study cannot be compared reliably over time. It was nevertheless found to be consistent with earlier research on fat consumption, fatty acid composition, and fruit and veg consumption in the 2003 study. Saturated fatty acids, fiber, salmon, fruit, and vegetables were much lower in the normal diet of a young adult in 2003 than they should have been.

How to Eat Healthier in 25 Easy Steps:

The Health Benefits of eating a diet high in fruits and vegetables, including a lower risk of chronic illness and overall physical health, have been scientifically proven.

Making significant dietary alterations, on the other hand, can be quite frightening.

Consider making only a few minor adjustments rather than a slew of more significant ones. When dealing with one problem at a time, it's a lot easier than trying to tackle all of them at once (Multari *et al.*, 2015).

These 25 easy tweaks may be made to any supper to make it healthier. Remember, you don't have to finish them all at once. It's also possible to gradually adjust to the new circumstances.

A person's weight gain risk might be determined by how rapidly they consume their meals. Fast eaters, on the other hand, consume more food and have a higher BMI than slow eaters, according to research. The quantity of food you consume and how satisfied you are with your meal are all controlled by hormones.

Whether an individual is hungry or full is transmitted to the brain through the release of hormones. It takes roughly 20 minutes for your brain to digest these instructions. As a consequence, eating slowly may allow your brain the time it needs to detect that you've eaten enough food to consume.

Several studies have shown that eating slowly can help you lose weight by lowering the number of calories you consume during meals. In addition to more complete chewing, slowing down eating is associated with improved weight control. Additionally, if you eat more slowly and frequently, you may consume less. If you enjoy refined bread, switch to whole-grain bread. Whole-grain bread may be simply changed for refined grain bread to enhance your diet. Refined grains have been related to a wide range of health concerns in several studies. Many health advantages, including decreased risk of type 2 diabetes, heart disease, and cancer have been associated with whole grains. They're also a fantastic source of fiber, B vitamins, and minerals like zinc, iron, magnesium, and manganese, to mention just a few (Lin et al., 2010).

In many circumstances, whole grain bread is preferable in flavor to refined bread. To confirm that your bread is produced entirely of whole grains rather than a combination of whole and refined grains, just check the label. Additionally, whole grains or nuts in the bread are helpful.

Take advantage of Greek yogurt. Compared to Greek yogurt, plain yogurt is lighter and creamier in texture.

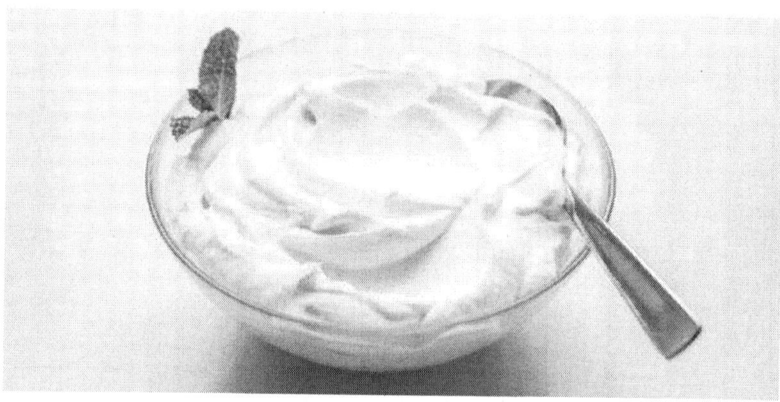

Figure 5.5: Greek yogurt.

To eliminate the extra whey or milk's watery component, it has been strained. Due to the greater fat and protein content, the end product is healthier than normal yogurt. In comparison to conventional yogurt, it provides up to 10 grams of protein every 3.5-ounce cup.

Fruits and vegetables are useful in dealing with problems with blood pressure. Among the dietary approaches to deal with hypertension have examined the effect on blood pressure of a diet rich in vegetables, fruits, and low-fat dairy products and restricted amounts of both saturated and total fat. Studies show that people with high blood pressure who followed this diet exhibited a reduction in systolic blood pressure by about 11 mm Hg. The same was exhibited in their diastolic blood pressure by almost 6 mm Hg as much as medications can achieve. A randomized trial referred to as the optimal macronutrient intake for heart health shows that the vegetable and fruit-rich diet causes a reduction in blood pressure, even more, when some carbohydrates are replaced with healthy unsaturated fat or protein. A meta-analysis of clinical trials and observational studies were done in 2014 showed that consumption of a vegetarian diet was linked to low blood pressure (Tang *et al.*, 2020).

Consumption of fruits and vegetables is also useful in preventing and treating cancer. Several early studies showed what appeared to be a strong link between eating vegetables and fruits and protection against cancer. Cohort studies are known to generally provide more reliable information compared to case-control studies. Cohort studies usually follow large groups of initially healthy individuals for years. Cohort studies usually don't rely on information from the past. Generally, data from cohort studies have not demonstrated that a diet rich in fruits and vegetables can prevent cancer.

A good example is a study done in the Nurses' Health Study and the Health Professionals Follow-up Study that occurred over a 14-year period which showed that women and men with the highest intake of vegetables and fruits were likely to develop cancer as those who ate the fewest daily servings. Another meta-analysis of cohort studies showed that consumption of large amounts of vegetables and fruits did not reduce the risk of death from cancer. This means that there is a possibility that certain types of vegetables and fruits could be useful in protecting against certain cancers. In other studies, it was noted that there are reduced risks of breast cancer among women who consume corn, grapes, bananas, and apples during adolescence and kale and oranges during early adulthood. Studies show that were was no protection for those who consume fruit juices at younger ages.

Fruits and vegetables are a great source of essential nutrients. This is because they act in concert and perform various roles in the body. They are used in shoring up bones, boosting our immune system, and healing wounds. They are at times involved in converting food into energy and repair of cellular damage. There are certain vitamins and minerals known to be found in some fruits and vegetables. It can be quite confusing to keep track of what vitamins and minerals do in the body. Examples of vitamins found in fruits and vegetables include Vitamin A, B, C, D, E, and K (Acosta-Estrada *et al.*, 2021).

Vegetables and fruits are rich in micronutrients. Macronutrients are nutrients needed by the body in small amounts. When the body suffers from a deficiency of macronutrients, it will suffer from diseases. Some of the diseases caused by the deficiency of vitamins include scurvy. Scurvy develops in a body that has not gotten any fresh fruits or vegetables known to be rich in vitamin C. The disease is characterized by listlessness of scurvy and bleeding gums. The deficiency of vegetables and fruits can also lead to blindness due to a deficiency of vitamin A found in fruits such as carrots.

The deficiency of vitamin D leads to rickets. Rickets is a condition characterized by soft weak bones that can lead to skeletal deformities such as bowed legs. To deal with this issue, the U.S has fortified milk with vitamin D. The deficiency of key micronutrients in the body can lead to substantial harm to the body while getting sufficient quantities can provide substantial benefit. Some of the benefits include strong bones where a combination of phosphorus, Magnesium, Vitamin K, vitamin D, and calcium are useful in protecting bones from fractures (Stintzing & Carle, 2004). Micronutrients in fruits and vegetables are useful in preventing birth defects such as brain and spinal birth defects in offspring. They also lead to healthy teeth. Minerals such as fluoride are useful in bone formation and keeping dental cavities from starting or worsening.

Vegetables and fruits are among the main ways through which minerals in soil find their way into the human body. Interactions between macronutrients are very important as they are useful. Vitamin D is useful in enabling the body pluck calcium from food sources passing through the digestive tract. Vitamin C facilitates the absorption of iron. It is important to note that the interplay of micronutrients is not always cooperative. Vitamin C is known to block the body's ability to assimilate copper as an essential mineral.

In fruits and vegetables, there are water-soluble vitamins. They are usually packed in watery portions of consumed foods. Such kinds of vitamins are usually absorbed into the bloodstream directly after digestion in the stomach. Our bodies are made of a large percentage of water. This allows the easy circulation of water-soluble vitamins in the body. The amount of water-soluble vitamins in the body is regulated continuously by our kidneys. Examples of water-soluble vitamins include B vitamins, Thiamin, Riboflavin, Pantothenic acid, Niacin, Folic acid, Biotin, Vitamin C, Vitamin B12, and Vitamin B6. There are various tasks done by water-soluble vitamins in the body. They include helping free energy found in consumed foods and keeping tissues healthy. With regards to releasing energy, several B vitamins are considered key components of certain coenzymes useful in releasing energy from food. Coenzymes are molecules that aid enzymes.

Under energy production, vitamins such as biotin, pantothenic acid, niacin, riboflavin, and thiamin are used. Vitamins B12, Vitamin B6, and folic acid i.e B9 are used in building proteins and cells. They facilitate the metabolism of amino acids which are the building blocks of proteins. They also facilitate cell multiplication. They are involved in the making of collagen (Shipp & Abdel-Aal, 2010). This usually involves vitamin C. It is known to knit together wounds, forming bases for teeth and bones and also supporting blood vessel walls. There are four fat-soluble vitamins. Sources for such vitamins are fatty food and oils. The body has fatty tissue which works alongside the liver to act as the main holding pen for vitamins. They release vitamins when needed.

This means that such vitamins can be thought of as time-release micronutrients. They can be consumed now and again in that they could be dosed weeks or months apart rather than daily. The excess is excreted by the body. There are fat-soluble vitamins namely Vitamin K, Vitamin D, Vitamin E, and Vitamin A. Altogether, the vitamin water helps keep the eyes, skin, lungs, nervous system, and gastrointestinal system in good repair. Some of the essential roles of these vitamins include building bones whereby in the absence of vitamins A, K, and D, the bone formation would not occur. They also protect vision. This mostly involves vitamin A which keeps eye cells healthy and protects our vision. These vitamins are also known to interact favorably allowing the body to absorb and store vitamin A. Water is an essential part of the diet as it facilitates digestion.

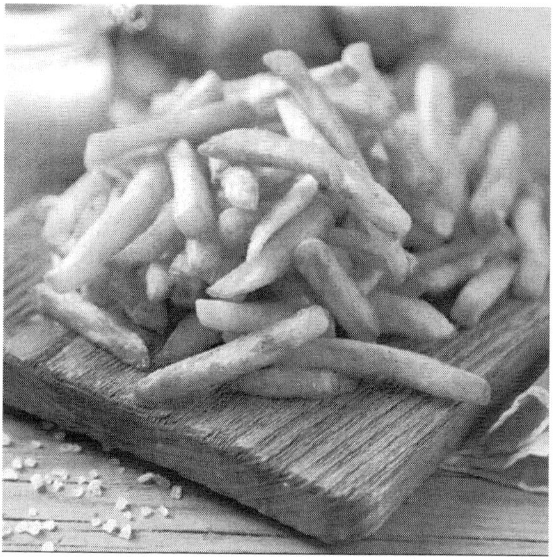

Figure 5.6: Deep-fried French fries.

- As a consequence, diabetics can manage their blood sugar levels more effectively in the short and long term.
- Rather than drinking your fruits, eat them.
- Fruits are high in nutrients such as water, fiber, vitamins, and antioxidants.
- According to one study, persons who ate a lot of fruits and vegetables were less likely to acquire heart disease, type 2 diabetes, and cancer (Kadam & Prabhasankar, 2010).
- Fruits' natural sugars are normally absorbed slowly and do not produce substantial rises in blood sugar levels since they include fiber and a range of plant components.
- Fruit juices, contrary to common perception, are not authorized.
- In many situations, concentrated fruit juice and sugar are utilized in the preparation of fruit juices instead of raw fruit. Some variants have the same amount of sugar as a sweet soft drink.
- Even the purest fruit juice lacks the fiber and chewing resistance supplied by entire fruits. As a result, fruit juice is more likely to increase your blood sugar, causing you to consume more in a single sitting.

- More time spent at home making meals
- Cooking at home rather than eating out is an excellent habit to develop.
- For starters, it is less costly.
- Cooking your meals is also a fantastic method to know precisely what you're putting into your body. There will be nothing hazardous or heavy in calories in your diet (Jacob et al., 2020).
- As long as you prepare enough food ahead of time, this provides a wholesome dinner the next day.
- Home cooking has been demonstrated to prevent obesity and offer a better diet overall in adolescents and teenagers.
- Increase the quantity of physical exercise you do.
- Regular physical exercise and a well-balanced diet have a high association. Regular physical activity can help to decrease or eliminate depression, stress, and other mental health disorders.
- These are the most prevalent sentiments related to binge eating and binge binging when it comes to emotional eating.
- Exercise can help you lose weight, boost energy, lessen your risk of chronic disease, and improve your sleep, in addition to strengthening your muscles and bones.
- When feasible, use the stairs or go for short walks, and aim for 30 minutes of moderate activity every day.
- Sparkling water should be used instead of sugar-sweetened drinks (Ibrahim et al., 2015).
- Sugar-sweetened sodas are one of the most harmful drinks you can ingest.
- Their high sugar content has been related to a variety of ailments, including heart disease, obesity, and type 2 diabetes.
- Furthermore, the extra sugar in these drinks has a distinct influence on appetite stimulation. Consuming fewer calories is insufficient to compensate for the calories previously consumed.
- Calories in a 16-ounce (492-mL) sweet drink: 207.
- Try a sugar-free choice or still or sparkling water instead of a sweet drink. Using this strategy, you will be able to lower your sugar and calorie intake.

- There should be no consumption of "diet" foods.
- Dietary supplement claims have a propensity to be incorrect or misleading. Because of their low-fat content, they Low-fat meals often have a greater sugar and calorie content than high-fat meals.
- Instead, choose whole meals such as fruits and vegetables.
- Make sure you receive a decent night's sleep.
- We can't emphasize how crucial it is to obtain a good night's sleep enough.
- Hunger levels rise as a result of sleep loss, which interferes with appetite regulation. Weight gain occurs as a result of an increase in calorie consumption.
- Those who do not get enough sleep, on the other hand, are more likely to be fat.
- Sleep deprivation has been demonstrated to have an impact on mood, memory, attention, and productivity, as well as athletic performance and glucose metabolism.
- Tobacco usage causes a variety of health issues, including inflammation and cardiovascular disease.
- Getting adequate quality sleep is so critical, and it's even better if you can do it all at once.
- Fresh berries are superior to dried fruit.
- Berries are a healthy snack option since they are high in vitamins, fiber, and antioxidants. For the great majority of items, fresh, frozen, or dry substitutes are easily available.
- Due to moisture are usually referred to as "fat-free," "low fat," "fat-reduced," or "low calorie."
- To compensate for the flavor and texture loss caused by fat, sugar and other flavor enhancers are routinely employed (Fabani et al., 2013).
    - loss, dried cultivars have a larger calorie and sugar content than fresh cultivars, although being equally healthy.
- A 3.5-ounce piece of fresh or frozen strawberries has 375 calories for every 100 grams of dried strawberries (Francesconi, 2007).
- Sugar increases the sugar content of dried fruits greatly, making them more caloric.

- Fresh fruit snacks are more delicious and contain fewer calories and sugar than pre-packaged competitors.
- Popcorn is a pleasant and healthful substitute for chips.
- Popcorn is a whole grain rich in vitamins, minerals, and fiber.
- In comparison to potato chips, which have 532 calories per 100-gram serving and only 3 grams of fiber, each 3.5-ounce serving of air-popped popcorn has 387 calories.
- A whole-grain diet reduces the risk of inflammation and cardiovascular disease, which is one of its many health advantages.
- Prepare your popcorn (not microwave popcorn) or buy air-popped popcorn for a healthy snack.
- Many commercially available kinds of popcorn, like potato chips, are high in fat, sugar, and salt.
- You should only utilize essential oils, which are extremely beneficial to your health.
- In recent decades, high-tech seed and vegetable oils have become an essential component of our diets.
- Soybean, cottonseed, sunflower, and canola oils are a few examples (Pop et al., 2019).
- These oils are high in omega-6 fatty acids, but low in omega-3 fatty acids, which are beneficial to the heart.

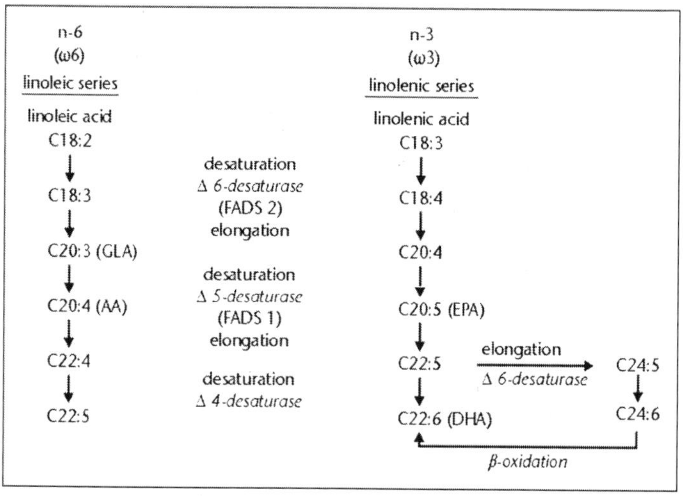

Omega-6 fatty acids.

- Chronic illnesses such as heart disease, cancer, and osteoporosis have been linked to an omega-6 to an omega-3 ratio greater than 2:1.
- Replace extra virgin olive oil, avocado oil, or coconut oil if you must use hazardous oil.
- Smaller dishes are used for meals.
- It has been proven that the size of your dinnerware influences how much food you consume.
- On a large dish, your portion will look smaller, whereas, on a small plate, it will appear greater.
- In one study, eating from a smaller plate was associated with higher feelings of fullness and lower energy intake in healthy persons (Odhaib et al., 2021).
- It's tough to compensate for overeating when you don't realize you've done it. To avoid overeating, use smaller plates to trick your brain into thinking you're eating more.
- Salad dressing should be served separately from the salad.
- For many people, being able to order a salad at a restaurant is a major accomplishment.
- Salads, on the other hand, do not have an ingredient list. Other salads on the menu are high in calories, in addition to the high-calorie dressing that smothers several salad dishes (such as the Caesar).
- It's simple to keep track of how much you're eating with the dressing on the side.
- Genuine coffee is the best way to consume stimulants.
- Coffee, one of the world's most popular beverages, has several health benefits.
- Its high antioxidant content has been linked to a lower risk of type 2 diabetes, cognitive decline, and liver disease, among other health benefits.
- Commercial coffee, on the other hand, is frequently loaded with sugars and sweeteners.
- The health benefits of coffee are quickly overwhelmed by the high sugar and calorie content when this kind of coffee is consumed (Murdoch et al., 2000).

- Sip your coffee decaffeinated or with a splash of milk or cream instead of sugar.
- Finally, making drastic dietary changes all at once may be detrimental.
- Consider some of the above-mentioned essential changes to get the most out of your diet.
- In addition to helping you manage portion sizes, these tactics can help you gain nutrients or acclimate to a new scenario.
- When these two factors are combined, you may have a healthy and sustainable diet without making major lifestyle changes.

5.14 8 Practical Tips Cover the Basics of Healthy Eating And Can Help You Make Healthier Choices

To maintain a good energy balance, your daily calorie intake should equal your daily workout. If you eat more calories than your body needs, the extra energy is stored as fat, resulting in weight gain. You will lose weight if you do not consume enough calories and drinks. The most effective way to ensure that your body obtains the nutrients it needed is to eat a variety of meals. A man's daily caloric intake should be around 2,500. Women should consume at least 2,000 calories each day to maintain a healthy weight. In the United Kingdom, the great majority of individuals consume more calories than they need (Multari *et al.,* 2015).

Consume a high proportion of starchy carbohydrates with high fiber content for the bulk of your meals. Starch-derived carbohydrates should not account for more than one-third of your overall calorie consumption. Potatoes, bread, rice, pasta, and cereals are among the items on the list. Whole-wheat pasta, brown rice, and skin-on potatoes are all high in fiber and whole grains and can be substituted for pasta. As a result, they have the potential to deliver more sustained energy than white or refined starchy carbs. Every main meal should include at least one starchy item. Even though starchy meals contain less than half the carbohydrate content of fat, some individuals feel they are oily. Reduce the amount of fat used in the preparation and presentation of these meals, such as oil on chips, butter on toast, and rich pasta sauces.

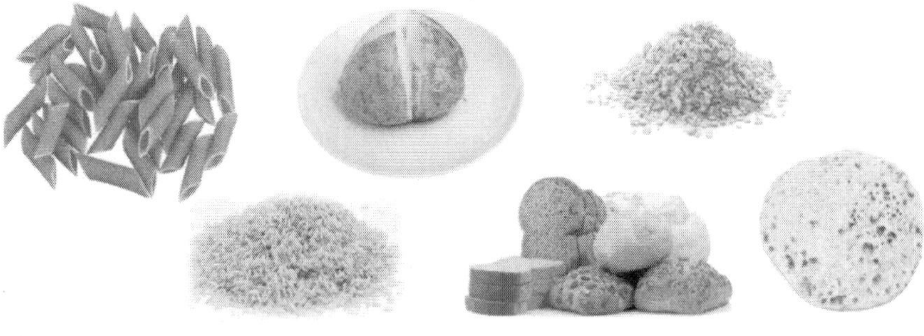

Figure 5.7: Starchy carbohydrates.

Consume a wide range of fruits and vegetables.

A person should eat at least five different fruits and vegetables every day. Fresh, frozen, tinned, dry, and juiced foods are also available. It is not nearly as tough as it looks to consume the required five servings of fruits and vegetables every day. Instead of sliced bananas, a piece of fresh fruit makes a fantastic mid-morning snack. Fruits and vegetables, whether fresh, canned, or frozen, weigh around 80 grams apiece. Dried fruit has around 30 grams of fiber per serving. A portion of fruit juice, vegetable juice, or smoothie is likewise regarded as 150 mL; however, owing to the high sugar content and danger of tooth damage, you should restrict yourself to one per day (Lin *et al.,* 2010).

Increase your intake of fish, especially fatty kinds.

- Aside from being a rich source of protein, fish is also high in a range of nutrients. At least two fish dinners each week are advised, one of which should be fatty. Oily fish contain omega-3 fatty acids, which may help lessen the risk of coronary heart disease.
- Oily fish, such as salmon and trout, as well as pilchards and mackerel, are high in omega-3 fatty acids.
- Haddock, plaice, coley, cod, tuna, skate, and hake are examples of non-oily fish.
- Remember that canned and smoked fish can have a high salt content, so keep this in mind while purchasing. Regardless of whether some fish species are in short supply, the great majority of people should increase their fish diet. Consumption of sugar and saturated fat should be decreased.

You need fat in your diet, but you must keep track of how much and what sort of fat you ingest. Safflower oil and coconut oil are examples of unsaturated fats. A diet heavy in saturated fat can elevate blood cholesterol levels, increasing your risk of heart disease. On average, males should consume no more than 30 grams of saturated fat each day. Women should limit their saturated fat consumption to no more than 20 grams per day. Children under the age of 11 should eat less saturated fat than adults, but they should not follow a low-fat diet. Saturated fat may be found in dairy items such as butter and hard cheeses, baked products such as cakes and cookies, as well as fatty cuts of meat and sausages (Linares et al., 2017). Reduce your diet of saturated fat and increase your intake of unsaturated fats, such as those found in vegetable oils and spreads, fatty fish, and avocados, to maintain a healthy weight. In place of butter, lard, or ghee, use a tiny quantity of vegetable or olive oil or a low-fat spread. Trim any visible fat from the meat before serving. Because of their high-calorie content, fats should be ingested in moderation.

Sugar

Regular use of sugary foods and beverages may contribute to obesity and tooth damage. Due to their caloric density, overconsumption of high-calorie, high-kilojoule sweet foods and beverages can result in weight gain. They can also cause tooth decay, especially if consumed between meals. Sugars added to meals or beverages, as well as sugars present naturally in honey, syrups, and unsweetened fruit juices and smoothies, are examples of free sugars. This sort of sugar, not the sugar found in fruits and milk, should be avoided.

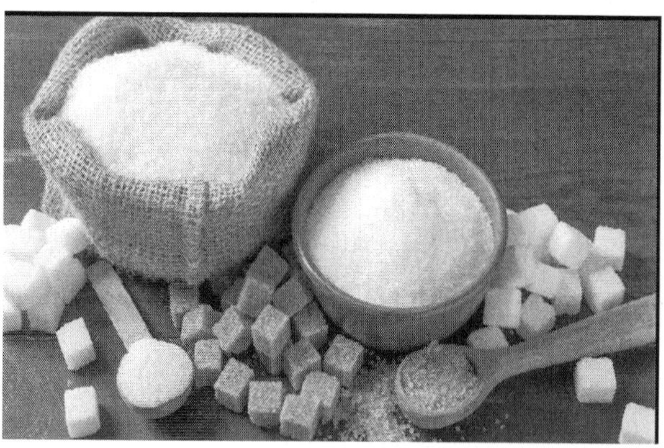

Figure 5.8: Sugar.

Sugars may be found in an extraordinarily wide range of packaged foods and drinks in their natural condition. Free sugars can be found in sugar-sweetened soft drinks, sugar-sweetened morning cereals, cakes, biscuits, pastries, and puddings, as well as candies, chocolate, and alcoholic beverages. Food labels can be beneficial. These may be used to calculate the sugar level of different foods. A high-sugar meal has at least 22.5 grams of total sugar per 100 grams, whereas a low-sugar meal has no more than 5 grams (Haque et al., 2020).

Salt consumption should be limited to no more than 6 grams per day.

Excessive salt consumption can cause blood pressure to increase. Individuals with high blood pressure are more likely to develop heart disease or have a stroke. Even if you don't add salt to your diet, you may eat too much salt. Breakfast cereals, soups, bread, and sauces account for around three-quarters of the salt you consume. Reading food labels might aid you in saving money. A food is deemed salty if it contains more than 1.5 grams of salt per 100 grams. Adults and children over the age of 11 should keep their daily salt consumption to no more than 6g (approximately a tablespoon). Children under the age of five should receive much less.

It is vital to maintain a healthy weight and engage in physical activity.

Regular exercise combined with a good diet can help you prevent significant health problems. It is also essential for general health and fitness. Obesity has been linked to several health issues, such as type 2 diabetes, some malignancies, cardiovascular disease, and stroke. Furthermore, being underweight is probably harmful to your health. The great majority of people want to reduce weight by limiting their calorie intake. Try consuming fewer calories and increasing your physical activity if you want to lose weight. Consuming a nutritious, well-balanced diet may make it simpler to maintain a healthy weight. Use the BMI healthy weight calculator to discover your current weight. Begin the NHS weight-loss program, which mixes nutrition and activity for 12 weeks. If you are underweight, please visit the section on underweight adults (López *et al.,* 2019). Consult your doctor or a dietitian if you are concerned about your weight.

Check to see whether you're thirsty.

Drink lots of water to avoid dehydration. The government recommended six to eight cups of coffee each day. Furthermore, this is in addition to fluids ingested during meals. While water, low-fat milk, and low-sugar liquids such as tea and coffee are not alcoholic, they are advised.

Carbonated beverages and soft drinks with added sugar are rich in calories and should be avoided. Furthermore, they may cause tooth injury. Even unsweetened fruit juices and smoothies have a lot of free sugar in them. You should not drink more than 150ml of fruit juice, vegetable juice, or smoothies each day (about one small glass). If the weather is hot or you're exercising, remind yourself to drink lots of water.

Breakfast is an essential meal that should not be skipped. Some people feel that missing breakfast can help them lose weight. A nutritious breakfast that is high in fiber and low in fat, sugar, and salt, on the other hand, can help you maintain a balanced diet and acquire the nutrients you need for maximum health. Using wholegrain reduced-sugar cereal, semi-skimmed milk, and fresh fruit, you can make a delicious and healthy meal.s

CHAPTER 6

HOW TO PROMOTE HEALTHY DIETS

CONTENTS

A healthy diet promotes or maintains good health. A balanced diet offers the body vital nutrients like fluid, macronutrients like protein, micronutrients like vitamins, and sufficient fiber and energy.

Fruits, vegetables, and grains are all part of a healthy diet, as are processed foods and sweetened beverages. A healthy diet can be made up of a diverse array of plant-based and animal-based foodstuffs, though vegans will need to supplement with a non-plant source of vitamin B12. Medical and government organizations publish a variety of nutrition guides to inform people about what they should eat to stay healthy. In some states, nutrition information labels are required to enable customers to choose between foods predicated on the constituents that are important to their health (Yousuf & Siddiqui, 2021).

6.1 RESEARCH

According to preliminary research, a diet rich in fruits and vegetables may reduce the risk of heart disease and mortality, but not cancer. For most people, proper nutrition and staying physically active can help them stay at a healthy weight and reduce their risk of obesity. In a scientific evaluation of the substantiation on diets for decreasing the risk of atherosclerosis published in 2021, it was discovered that:

"Atherosclerosis risk is reduced by consuming less salt and animal-derived foods and eating more plant-based foods like whole grains, fruits, vegetables, legumes, and nuts." The same can be said for substituting olive oil as well as other unsaturated-fat-rich oils for butter and another animal/tropical fats. [...] In terms of meat, new evidence distinguishes processed and red meat, both of which are linked to an increased risk of cardiovascular disease, from poultry, which has a CVD-neutral relationship for moderate intakes. [...] Most high glycemic index (GI) foods should be replaced with whole grain and low GI cereal foods, according to new research."

So far beyond a particular spectrum of illnesses, scientific research is looking into the effects of nutrition on health and lifespans. According to research, vastly increased conformity to Mediterranean diet configurations is linked to lower cumulative and cause-specific mortality, as well as longer health and lifespan (Walker et al., 2015). The strongly recommended constituents of the Mediterranean diet are being identified through research. It has a lot of similarities to the Okinawa diet, which is also very healthy. Various nutrients' potential anti-aging mechanisms are still unknown.

According to studies, dietary adjustments are a major contributor to national relative increases in life expectancy.

6.2 EXTENDING YOUR LIFE

The concept of life extension is to prolong the human lifespan, either moderately through medical advancements or significantly by boosting the maximum lifespan beyond the currently accepted limit of 125 years.

Numerous researchers in the field, as well as "life extensionists," "immortalists," and "longevists" (those who want to live longer lives), believe that future advancements in cellular rejuvenation, stem cells, regenerative medical treatments, molecular restoration, genetic manipulation, pharmaceuticals, and organ replacement (including with synthetic organs or xenotransplantations) will ultimately enable humans to live indefinitely (Vanbergen & Initiative, 2013). Bioethicists are debating the ethical implications of life extension if it becomes a reality.

The sale of ostensibly anti-aging products like supplements and hormone replacement is a multibillion-dollar global business. In the United States, for instance, the industry that endorses the prescribing of hormones as a therapy to slow or counteract the aging process yielded about $50 billion in revenue in 2009. However, the efficacy and safety of these hormone products have yet to be established.

During the aging process, an organism's macromolecules, cells, tissues, and organ systems accrue damage. "Genetic changes, telomere attrition, epigenetic variations, the decline of proteostasis, deregulated nutrient detecting, mitochondrial abnormalities, cellular senescence, stem cell depletion, and affected intercellular communication" are all thought to contribute to aging. Free radical-induced oxidation harm to cell components is considered to lead to aging too.

The longest recorded human lifespan is 122 years and 164 days, in the particular instance of Jeanne Calment, who'd been born in 1875 and died in 1997, as per records, while the limited lifespan of a wildtype mouse, which is frequently used as a model in aging studies, is around three years. Variations in the system performance of Gene regulation, antioxidant countermeasures, energy metabolism, proteostasis maintenance, and material recovery processes like autophagy may explain the differences in aging rates in both humans and mice (Acosta-Estrada *et al.*, 2021).

Infant and child mortality, which is regularly associated with infectious diseases or nutritional problems, reduces a population's average life expectancy. Accidental death and age-related chronic diseases, like cancer or cardiovascular disease, play a significant role in mortality as people get older. Enhanced medical care, vaccinations, a healthy diet, exercise, and the avoidance of risks like smoking can all help to extend one's expected lifespan.

The rate of aging in a species' genes, as well as external conditions, establish its maximum lifespan. Caloric constraints, gene manipulation, and pharmaceutical administration are all well-known procedures for prolonging maximum lifespan in model organisms like nematodes, fruit flies, and mice. Another method involves applying evolutionary forces like breeding only older members or changing extrinsic mortality levels. Hydra, planarian flatworms, as well as certain sponges, corals, and jellyfish, for example, do not die of old age and have the potential to live forever.

6.3 SUPPLEMENTS AND DIETS

6.3.1 Antioxidants and Vitamins

According to the free-radical theory of aging, antioxidant supplements may help people live longer. Supplementing with vitamin A (as -carotene) and vitamin E, on the other hand, has been linked to an increased risk of death in studies. In other studies, there was no link between vitamin E as well as other vitamins and mortality (Ambuja & Rajakumar, 2018).

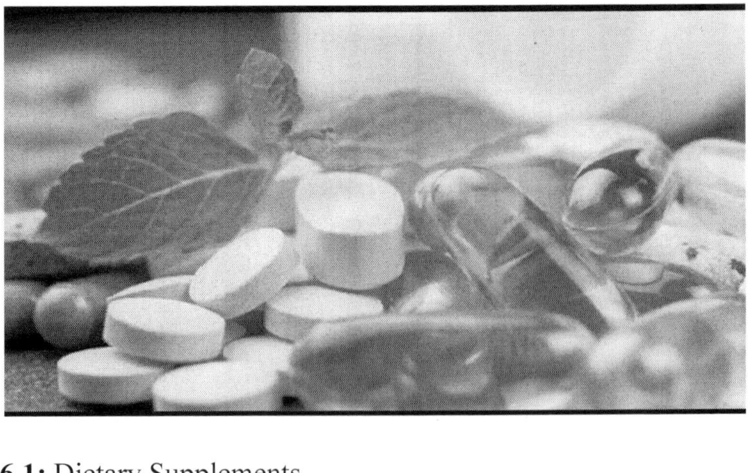

Figure 6.1: Dietary Supplements.

6.3.2 Dietary Restriction

Calorie restriction has been demonstrated to prolong the lives of mice, yeast, and rhesus monkeys in some studies. However, calorie restriction did not enhance survival in rhesus monkeys in a more recent study. The long-term health impacts of reasonable caloric restriction combined with adequate nutrition in humans are unknown.

As per two scientific evaluations published in 2021, growing evidence suggests that dietary restriction (DR) – primarily intermittent fasting and caloric restriction – causes most of the same favorable variations in human adults as it does in researched organisms, possibly extending health and lifespan further than the benefits of healthy body weight. Which DR protocols and combinations are beneficial or most efficient in humans is widely undefined and is currently being investigated. A new geroscience field called "precision nutrigeroscience" is postulated, which takes into account the possibility of nutritional intervention modifications per person (e.g. due to differences in genetics and age). Intermittent fasting alludes to periods when no food is consumed and only water or tea/coffee is consumed – for example, a timeframe of daily time-restricted consumption with a window of 8 to 12 hours for any caloric intake – and can be coupled with overall caloric restriction and different versions of the Mediterranean diet, that are known to have long-term cardiovascular and longevity advantages (Turner & Thompson, 2013).

Greater protein consumption "may be needed to increase muscle preservation in lean, resistance-trained participants" during intervals of caloric limitation, and "resistance training (RT) can reduce muscle loss throughout caloric restriction," with strength training also being linked to a "10–17 percent reduced risk of all-cause death rates, cardiovascular disease (CVD), total cancer, diabetes, and lung cancer."

AMPK, mTOR, insulin-related pathways, sirtuins, NAD+, NFkB, and FOXO, as well as, by extension, processes like autophagy, have all been implicated in the health advantages of caloric restriction and methionine-reduction/restriction. Healthy Diet

According to research, growing conformity to Mediterranean diet styles is linked to lower cumulative and cause-specific mortality, as well as longer health and lifespan. The vital beneficial elements of the Mediterranean diet are being identified through research. It has a lot of similarities to the Okinawa diet, which is also very healthy. Various nutrients' potential anti-aging mechanisms are still unknown.

According to studies, lifestyle modifications are a major contributor to national relative increases in life expectancy.

6.3.3 Microbiome

Mechanistically, studies suggest that the gut microenvironment, which differs from person to person and changes over time, is also involved in the beneficial effects. As a result, various diet supplements with prebiotics, differing probiotics and synbiotics, and fecal microbiome composition transplantation are being evaluated for life extension, primarily for extending healthspan, with many important questions still unanswered (Ballester-Sánchez *et al.*, 2019).

An ideal diet:

The following are some methods for developing optimal diets for health and longevity:

- Modifying or further particularizing the Mediterranean diet as a benchmark, for example, by adding various foods thought to be healthy (e.g., due to findings of various mechanistic impacts) to the regular diet, or by increasing plant-based (but protein-rich) foods coupled with extensive restriction of red meat consumption and regular reasonable consumption of green tea or coffee while maintaining sufficient calcium intake, or by incorporating additional foods considered to be healthy (e.g., due to findings regarding various mechanistic impacts) to the regular diet.
- Using the currently offered meta-analyses and data from mostly epidemiological studies to infer an ideal diet for all levels and types of physical activities, age, and other personal characteristics. This was done for an instrument and infographics that show the comparative overall life extension possibilities of various food groups in different populations, suggesting, for instance, a 20-year-old European male having switched to the "optimal diet" could acquire an average of 13.7 years of life, while a 60-year-old female making the switch to the "optimal diet" in the United States could attain an average of 8.0 years of life. Extra legumes, whole grains, and nuts, as well as less red and processed meat, were found to provide the greatest benefits. Sugar-sweetened beverages are not allowed in the optimized diet (shifting from a "standard American diet" of 500 grams per day to 0 grams per

day). The impact of eggs, white meat, and oils, personal alteration in potential risk factors, unknowns for future advancement of clinical treatments, and lifestyle changes, according to the study, are all unclear (Tang *et al.,* 2020).

6.4 DIET AND CANCER

Dietary factors are known to have a significant impact on cancer risk, with various dietary aspects either raising or lowering risk. Lack of physical activity likely contributes to a 7% risk of cancer occurrence, while diet and obesity may be linked to 30-35 percent of cancer deaths. According to a review published in 2011, total caloric intake has an impact on cancer incidence and progression.

Whereas many dietary guidelines have been postulated to reduce cancer risk, only a few have substantial scientific evidence to back them up. Obesity and alcohol consumption have been linked to the occurrence and progression of certain cancers. Reduced consumption of sugar-sweetened beverages is suggested as a means to combat obesity (Stintzing & Carle, 2004). A diet high in red meat and low in fruits and vegetables has been suggested but not proven, and the effect may be minor in well-nourished individuals who preserve a healthy weight.

Some foods have been linked to certain cancers. Eating red or processed meat has been associated with a greater risk of breast cancer, colon cancer, prostate cancer, and pancreatic cancer in research findings, which could be clarified in portion by the existence of carcinogens in foods cooked at extreme temperatures. Aflatoxin B1, a common food contaminant, raises the risk of liver cancer, whereas coffee consumption lowers the risk. Chewing betel nuts causes oral cancer. Because of its high salt diet, stomach cancer is more prevalent in Japan. Immigrant communities are more prone to developing the risks of their new nation within one generation, implying a significant link between diet and cancer.

Weight control and eating "primarily vegetables, fruit, whole grains, and fish, with a lowered intake of red meat, animal fat, and processed sugar" are common cancer-prevention dietary recommendations.

6.5 RESTRICTIVE DIETS

A variety of diets and nutrition-based regimens have been claimed to be effective in the fight against cancer. The Breuss diet, Gerson therapy, the

Budwig protocol, and the macrobiotic diet are all popular "anti-cancer" diets. None of these diets have been proven to work, and some have even been demonstrated to be harmful (Bulaj *et al.,* 2016).

6.5.1 Dietary Habits

Multi-variate statistics, like principal components assessment and factor analysis, are used by nutritional epidemiologists to determine how trends in dietary behavior impact the risk of getting cancer. (The Mediterranean diet is the most researched dietary pattern.) Epidemiologists divide people into quantiles predicated on their diet quality score. They measure the relationship between observed values and the propagation of cancer prevalence (in case of reports) and cancer incidence to analyze the influence of dietary habits on cancer risk (in longitudinal studies). Other factors are commonly included in their statistical theory to account for other discrepancies between cancer patients and non-cancer patients (confounders). In the case of breast cancer, there is a consistent trend that women who eat a more "sensible or healthy" diet, i.e. a diet rich in fruits and vegetables, have a lower risk of developing the disease. A "drinker dietary pattern" is also linked to an increased risk of breast cancer, whereas there is no link between a more "western" diet and an increased risk of breast cancer (Cassani *et al*., 2020). Pickled foods have been linked to the development of cancer.

6.5.2 Alcohol

A handful of cancers have been linked to the consumption of alcohol. Alcohol is responsible for 3.6 percent of all cancer cases and 3.5 percent of cancer deaths worldwide. Alcohol consumption is linked to breast cancer in women. Alcohol also raises the risk of mouth, esophageal, pharyngeal, and laryngeal cancers, as well as colorectal cancer, liver cancer, stomach cancer, and ovarian cancer. Alcohol is classified as a Group 1 carcinogen by the World Health Organization's International Agency for Research on Cancer. According to its assessment, "There is substantial proof that alcoholic beverages cause cancer in humans. People are carcinogenic to alcoholic beverages."

6.5.3 Processed Meats

The World Health Organization's International Agency for Research on Cancer reported in 2015 that consuming processed meat (e.g., bacon, ham, hot dogs, sausages) or red meat was associated with certain cancers.

6.5.4 Fruits and Vegetables, as well as Fiber

The findings on the impact of dietary fiber on colon cancer risk are varied, with certain forms of evidence indicating an advantage and others indicating a lack of benefit. While eating fruits and vegetables has health benefits, it has a lower impact on cancer prevention than previously thought. Phytoestrogens are abundant in soy. Phytoestrogens are naturally occurring substances with weak estrogenic effects (Shipp & Abdel-Aal, 2010).

High fiber intake was linked to a lower risk of premenopausal and postmenopausal breast cancers, as well as an elevated survival rate in breast cancer patients, according to two meta-analyses published in 2020.

Fruit, but not vegetables, were found to protect against upper gastrointestinal tract cancer in a recent study. While fruits, vegetables, and fiber helped to prevent colorectal cancer, fiber helped to prevent liver cancer.

6.5.5 Flavonoids

"The most prevalent group of polyphenolic substances in the human diet and are detected ubiquitously in plants," according to Flavonoids (particularly flavonoids like catechins). While some research findings have posited that flavonoids may help prevent cancer, others have been ambiguous or have suggested that they may be damaging.

6.5.6 Mushrooms

"At this time, there is no scientific proof that any kinds of mushroom or mushroom extract can preclude or cure cancer," as per Cancer Research UK, through research into some organisms.

- According to the American Cancer Society, there is no compelling proof that soy products have anticancer properties.
- Drinking green tea does not affect the risk of cancer.
- Women and men who drank coffee had a reduced risk of liver cancer, according to a meta-analysis published in 2016. Coffee was associated with decreased risk of liver and endometrial cancer, according to a meta-analysis review (Sharma *et al.*, 2021).
- According to a systematic review published in 2014, "there is no concrete proof that vitamin D supplementation reduces the risk of cancer in primarily elderly community-dwelling women."

6.6 FOOD PYRAMID

A food pyramid depicts the ideal serving size for every other of the basic food groups to consume each day. In 1974, Sweden released the first pyramid. The "Food Guide Pyramid" or "Eating Right Pyramid" was presented by the United States Department of Agriculture (USDA) in 1992. It was renamed "MyPlate" in 2011 after being updated to "MyPyramid" in 2005 (Rochfort, 2005).

In 1972, Sweden's National Board of Health and Welfare came up with the concept of "basic foods," which were both inexpensive and nutritious, and "supplemental foods," which provided nutrition not found in the basic foods. The following year, Anna-Britt Agnsäter, the head of Kooperativa Förbundet's "test kitchen," did a presentation on how to depict these food groups. Fjalar Clemes, one of the attendees, proposed a triangle with basic foods at the bottom. Agnsäter developed the concept into the first food guide pyramid, which was first published in KF's Vi magazine in 1974. The pyramid was partitioned into three sections: basic foods at the bottom, such as milk, cheese, margarine, bread, cereals, and potato; supplemental vegetables and fruit in the middle; and supplemental meat, fish, and eggs at the top. The pyramid battled with the National Board's "dietary circle," which KF criticized for mirroring a seven-slice cake and failing to specify how much of each food should be consumed. KF continued to endorse the pyramid even as the Board detached itself from it.

Other Northern European countries, and also West Germany, Japan, and Sri Lanka established food pyramids. In 1992, the United States created its first food pyramid.

Depending on meta-analysis, the World Health Organization and the Food and Agriculture Organization established recommendations that can be successfully symbolized in a food pyramid on priorities to prevent obesity, poor nutrition, chronic diseases, and dental caries, though they present it as a table rather than a "pyramid." The design is similar to the USDA food pyramid in some ways, but there are important differences between types of fats and a more striking distinction between free sugars and sugars in their organic state when it comes to carbohydrates (Caporgno & Mathys, 2018).

Because of their impact on the intended concerns that the "pyramid" is aimed at correcting, some food substances have been highlighted. Nevertheless, in a later revision, some guidelines are removed because they are invariably followed by others, while some other sub-categories are introduced.

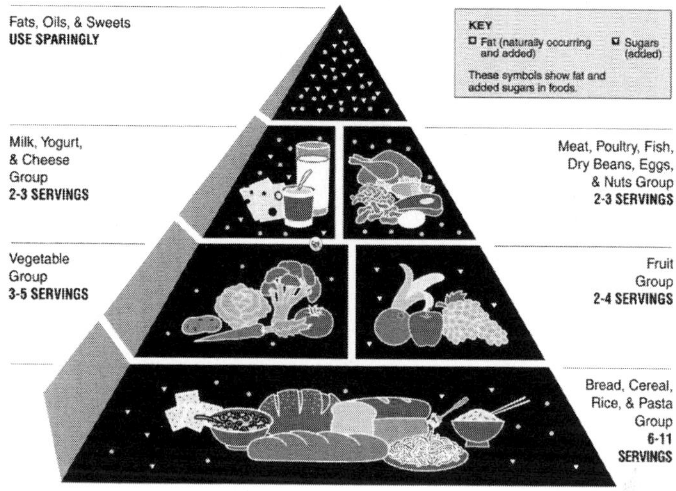

Figure 6.2: The USDA's original food pyramid, from 1992 to 2005.

6.6.1 Vegetables

A vegetable is a savory but not sweet part of a plant that is consumed by humans. Vegetables are not grains, fruits, nuts, spices, or herbs. The stem, root, flower, and other parts of the plant, for instance, can be eaten as vegetables. Vegetables are high in vitamins and minerals, but different vegetables have different micronutrient balances, so it's important to eat a variety of them (Ribeiro et al., 2019). Vitamin A is found in oranges and dark green vegetables, vitamin C is found in dark green vegetables, and iron and calcium are found in broccoli and related plants. Vegetables are low in fats and calories, but the ingredients used to prepare them can often increase these.

6.6.2 Grains

When unrefined, these foods offer complex carbohydrates, which are a rich source of energy and nutrition. Maize, wheat, pasta, and rice are just a few examples.

6.6.3 Fruits

Fruits are the sweet-tasting seed-bearing sections of plants, or every once in a while sweet parts of plants that do not hold seeds, in regards to food (instead of botany). Apples, oranges, grapes, bananas, and other fruits fall into this category. Fruits are a good source of organic sugars, fiber, and vitamins while being low in calories and fat. Fruit processing, such as canning or making juice, can result in the addition of sugars and the removal of nutrients. The fruit and vegetable food groups are sometimes mixed. Note that a large number of plant species generate seed pods that are presumed fruits in botany, and that some botanical fruits, such as tomatoes and avocados, are traditionally not deemed "fruits" in gastronomy since they have little or no distinctive sweet taste.

6.6.4 Dairy

Dairy products are made from the milk of mammals, most commonly cattle, but not always. Milk, yogurt, and cheese are among them. Milk and its derivatives are high in calcium, protein, phosphorus, vitamin A, and vitamin D, as well as other nutrients. However, when compared to vegetables, fruits, and whole grains, several more dairy products are full of saturated fat and cholesterol, which is why skimmed items are produced as an option (Raes et al., 2004). Adults were once encouraged to drink three cups of dairy products each day. More recently, evidence has accumulated that dairy products have more adverse health effects than originally believed, as well as fewer benefits.

Current findings, for instance, have found no link between dairy products and bone strength or fewer fractures; on the other hand, another analysis revealed that milk (and yogurt) consumption leads to higher bone mineral density in the hip. All in all, the majority of studies imply that dairy has some benefits for bone health, owing to the other nutrients found in milk.

6.6.5 Meat and Beans

Meat is an animal's tissue, usually muscle, which is consumed by humans. There is a wide variety of meats available because most parts of several animals are nutritious. Meat is a good source of protein, iron, zinc, and vitamin B12, among other nutrients. Beef, chicken, pork, fish, shrimp, and eggs are examples of meats, poultry, and fish.

The meat association is one of the food guide pyramid's most compressed food groups. Because many of the same nutrients encountered in meat can also be observed in foods such as eggs, dry beans, and nuts, these foods are often classified as meat alternatives. Tofu, products that closely mimic meat or fish and yet are made from soy, eggs, and cheeses are examples (Proksch et al., 2003).

Meat analogs, tofu, beans, lentils, chickpeas, nuts, and other high-protein vegetables are also fitted in this collection for those who do not eat meat or animal products. Adults should eat 2–3 servings per day, according to the food pyramid. Approximately the size of a stack of cards, one serving of meat is 4 oz (110 g).

6.6.6 Oils and Sweets

Because the tip of a food pyramid is the tiniest part, the fats and sweets at the top of the Food Pyramid must account for the tiniest percentage of the diet. The foods at the top of the food pyramid must be consumed in moderation because they are high in calories but low in nutrition. Salad dressings, oils, cream, butter, margarine, sugars, fizzy drinks, sweets, and sugary desserts are among these foods. The fat ring and sugar triangle on the 1992-2005 pyramid are strewn about to depict naturally found fats and sugars in different foods.

Because there is plenty of fat and sugar in the remainder of the diet, the purpose is to minimize the urge to eat too much junk food and inordinate fats and sugars. The triangles in the Fruit Group, for instance, refer to the fact that sugar is an unavoidable part of that group.

6.7 CONTROVERSY

Certain dietary selections related to heart disease, including a daily serving of 8 oz (230 g) hamburger, were theoretically allowed under the pyramid. Inside the protein-rich group, the pyramid also had little differentiation ("Meat, Poultry, Fish, Dry Beans, Eggs, and Nuts").

The United States Department of Agriculture (USDA) stopped the public release of its Eating Right Pyramid in 1991, following complaints from meat and dairy special interests groups about the guide's depiction of their products. Notwithstanding the USDA's interpretations that the guide needed more development and experiments, the Eating Right Pyramid was not announced officially until a year later, after its material had been confirmed by additional research (Dayan et al., 2009). Even the typography of the manual was changed this time to placate industry fears. This was just one of many instances wherein the food industry tried to challenge federal dietary guidelines to benefit their bottom line.

Some of the old pyramid's recommended quantities for various types of food have also been criticized for their lack of clarity. For example, the protein-rich group is recommended for two to three servings, but this is meant to be a maximum. The pyramid suggests two to four servings of fruit, but this is the bare minimum.

The fats group has been placed at the very top of the pyramid, with the instruction to enjoy as little as feasible, which some have found to be controversial. The guide advises people to eat as little fat as reasonably practicable, which can lead to health issues because fat is necessary for overall health. According to research, unsaturated fats can help you lose weight, reduce your risk of heart disease, lower your blood sugar, or even lower your cholesterol. They're also very long-lasting and help maintain blood sugar levels stable. Furthermore, these fats are beneficial to brain function.

According to several books, food and agricultural affiliations wield undue political influence over the USDA. Food companies, like milk producers, have been accused of bribing the US Department of Agriculture to increase the size of the colored areas on the recently founded food pyramid for their specific product. The milk segment of the pyramid is said to be the simplest to observe out of the six, leading people to believe that more milk should indeed be ingested daily than the others.

Moreover, the integration of milk as a distinct food group presupposes that it is an important component of a healthy diet, even after the fact that many people are lactose intolerant or select to avoid dairy, and a proportion of cultures have traditionally ingested little or no milk products. In his book Eat to Live, Joel Fuhrman claims that taxpayers in the United States must pay $20 billion in price controls to artificially drop the cost of livestock feed to support the dairy, beef, and veal enterprises, and then pay the medical expenses for overweight demography (Pop et al., 2019). He wonders if the USDA is influenced by the food industry since a scientifically based food pyramid would include vegetables as the framework.

These disagreements prompted the establishment of tailor made pyramids, e.g. a Vegetarian Diet Pyramids.

6.8 WORLD HEALTH ORGANIZATION

With regard to both populations and individuals, the World Health Organization (WHO) tends to make the mentioned five recommendations:

- Eat approximately the same amount of calories as your body uses to maintain a healthy weight.

- Consume fats in moderation. Fats should account for no more than 30% of total calories. Unsaturated fats are preferable to saturated fats. Trans fats should be avoided.
- Every day, consume at least 400 grams of fruits and vegetables (potatoes, sweet potatoes, cassava, and other starchy roots do not count). Legumes (e.g. lentils, beans), whole grains, and nuts are all part of a healthy diet (Odhaib et al., 2021).
- Keep simple sugars to less than 10% of your total calorie intake (below 5 percent of calories or 25 grams maybe even better).
- Limit salt/sodium intake from all sources and use iodized salt. A daily salt intake of fewer than 5 grams can lower the risk of cardiovascular disease.

According to the WHO, 2.8 percent of deaths worldwide are caused by a lack of vegetables and fruits.

WHO recommendations are as follows:

- going to ensure that the foods selected contain adequate amounts of vitamins and minerals;
- avoiding substances that are directly toxic (e.g. heavy metals) or carcinogenic (e.g. benzene);
- avoiding human pathogen-contaminated foods (e.g., E. coli, tapeworm eggs);
- and substituting polyunsaturated fats for saturated fats in the diet to lower the risk of coronary heart disease and diabetes (Da Silva *et al*., 2016).

A nutritious diet can help prevent malnutrition in all of its forms, as well as a variety of noncommunicable diseases (NCDs) and other illnesses. However, dietary patterns have shifted as a consequence of the enhanced manufacturing of processed foods, fast urbanization, and changing consumer preferences. People are eating more foods high in energy, fats, free sugars, and salt/sodium, and so many people are not eating enough fruit, vegetables, and whole grains.

Diet is influenced by a person's food preferences, as well as the accessibility and affordability of nutritious foods, as well as socio-cultural factors. As a result, promoting a healthy food environment necessitates collaboration from a variety of sectors and interested parties, such as the government, the public sector, and the private sector.

Governments play a critical role in fostering healthy food surroundings that makes it simple for people to adopt and preserve healthy eating habits. Policymakers can take the following steps to add value:

- Aligning trade, food system, and agricultural regulations with public health protection and promotion (Murdoch *et al*., 2000);
- Increasing interest in healthy foods and meals among consumers; and
- Encouraging healthy eating habits throughout one's life.

The World Health Assembly adopted the WHO Global Strategy on Diet, Physical Activity, and Health in 2004. It urged governments, the World Health Organization, worldwide partners, the private sector, and civil society to endorse nutritious foods and regular exercise at the global, regional, and local levels.

6.9 UNITED STATES DEPARTMENT OF AGRICULTURE

The United States Department of Agriculture's (USDA) Dietary Guidelines for Americans suggests three healthy diet trends for a 2000-calorie diet.

The guidelines place a strong emphasis on both health and ecological sustainability, as well as adaptability. It was written by the committee that drafted it: "The researchers discovered that a diet rich in plant-based foods, like vegetables, fruits, grains, legumes, nuts, and seeds, and low in calories and animal-based foods is much more health-promoting and has a lower carbon footprint than the existing American diet (Multari et al., 2015). This feeding trend can be implemented in many ways, including the "Healthy U.S.-style Pattern," "Healthy Vegetarian Pattern," and "Healthy Mediterranean-style Pattern."

Unless otherwise stated, food group quantities are per day.

The USDA's nutrition guidelines have a long history, with over 100 years of nutrition advice (United States Department of Agriculture). Over time, the recommendations have been revised to incorporate new research facts and public-health marketing practices. Dietary Guidelines for Americans 2015–2020 are the current recommendations. They've gone from four to eleven food groups over time. Various recommendations have been critiqued for not properly assessing scientific data about dietary modification and for being swayed by the agricultural sectors that the USDA supports.

Dr. Wilbur Olin Atwater published the USDA's first nutrition guidelines as a farmers' bulletin in 1894. Atwater advocated variety, proportionality, and moderation in his 1904 publication Principles of Nutrition and Nutritive Value of Food, as well as calorie counting and an effective, reasonably priced diet that centered on nutrient-rich foods and less fat, sugar, and starch. This knowledge existed before the finding of independent vitamins in 1910.

In 1916, nutritionist Caroline Hunt published Food for Young Children, which divided foods into five categories: milk and meat, cereals, vegetables and fruits, fats and fatty foods, sugars, and sugary foods, and fats and fatty foods. These five food groups were promoted to adults in 1917 in How to Select Food, and the recommendations continued to exist through the 1920s. In reaction to the Great Depression, the USDA presented four different food strategies in 1933 (Dixon & Sumner, 2003).

The first Recommended Dietary Allowances were published in 1941, outlining precise calorie, protein, iron, calcium, and vitamin A, B1, B2, B3, C, and D intakes.

The USDA's Center for Nutrition Policy and Promotion's current nutrition guide, MyPlate, is based on the Dietary Guidelines for Americans and provides a recommendation. In 2011, it supplemented the USDA's MyPyramid guide, marking the end of 19 years of USDA food pyramid illustrations. In the United States, MyPlate is expressed on food packaging and is used in nutrition education. A place designed set with a plate and glass split into 5 food groups that are suggested as part of a healthy diet is depicted in the graphic (Fabani et al., 2013). This diet plan includes a well-balanced mix of fruits, vegetables, grains, protein, and dairy. It is intended to serve as a guideline for Americans to use as a basis for making informed food choices. ChooseMyPlate.gov contains various types of these 5 subgroups predicated on a person's level of physical activity and personal attributes.

6.10 MYPLATE

The USDA's latest nutrition guide is called MyPlate. Dr. Wilbur Olin Atwater published the USDA's first dietary guidelines as a farmers' bulletin in 1894. Since then, the USDA has produced several public nutrition guides, including the Basic 7 (1943–1956), the Basic Four (1956–1992), the Food Guide Pyramid (1992–2005), and MyPyramid (2005–2013), among others. The USDA created MyPlate in 2011 to combine the recommendations of previous nutrition guides into an easy-to-read graphic.

Nutritional guides have been developed by some other governments and organizations. Plate diagrams are also used in some systems, such as the Eatwell Plate in the United Kingdom, the Australian Guide to Healthy Eating, and the American Diabetes Association's Create Your Plate system. The US Department of Agriculture announced plans to change the MyPlate constraints on milk, sodium, school breakfast, and school lunch possible alternatives in December 2018. Current nutritional research is producing new daily intake suggestions, which the USDA has been incorporating into newer MyPlate adjustments.

MyPlate is partitioned into four sections with roughly 30% grains, 40% vegetables, 10% fruits, and 20% protein, with a smaller circle portraying dairy, like a glass of milk or a yogurt cup (Linares *et al.,* 2017).

"Make 1/2 your plate fruits and vegetables," "Switch to 1 percent or skim milk," "Make at least half your grains whole," and "Vary your protein food choices" are among the additional recommendations on MyPlate. Portion regulation while still eating mindfully, as well as sodium and sugar cutbacks, are also recommended in the guidelines.

One of the key suggestions introduced through MyPlate's design is to make half of your plate fruits and vegetables. Many Americans do not ingest the recommended amount of fruits and vegetables or do not ingest a wide range of this food group. Because of the associated health benefits, the 2010 Dietary Guidelines suggest increasing fruit and vegetable consumption. Vitamin C, dietary fibers, and other vitamins and minerals are abundant in fruits and vegetables (López et al., 2019). These nutrients have also been linked to many health benefits, including the prevention of several diseases, the promotion of healthy aging, and the reduction of the risk of some cancers. Because of the numerous health advantages linked with fruits and vegetables, MyPlate encourages people to make this food group half of their plate.

MyPlate emphasizes the importance of including fruits and vegetables in one's diet because of the nutritive value they provide. To get the most nutrients, this nutritional suggestion suggests eating a multitude of both of these food groups. To get the most vitamins and minerals, MyPlate recommends eating a variety of fruits and vegetables in different colors.

First Lady Michelle Obama said at the launch of MyPlate, "Parents don't have time to measure out three ounces of chicken or look up the amount of rice or broccoli in a serving. We do, however, have time to examine our children's plates. And as long as they're consuming appropriate portions, with fruits and vegetables accounting for half of their meal along with lean proteins, whole grains, and low-fat dairy, we'll be fine. That's all there is to it."

Michelle Obama's Let'sMove! initiative has aimed MyPlate icon as a favorable nutritional framework to aid in the reduction of national obesity trends. The main goal of the Let'sMove Initiative is to give children a healthy life in an attempt to generate a healthier society in the long term (Karioti *et al.*, 2015). Michelle Obama's action plan has chosen to advertise MyPlate and ChooseMyPlate.gov to help achieve the overall goal of reducing obesity in the United States.

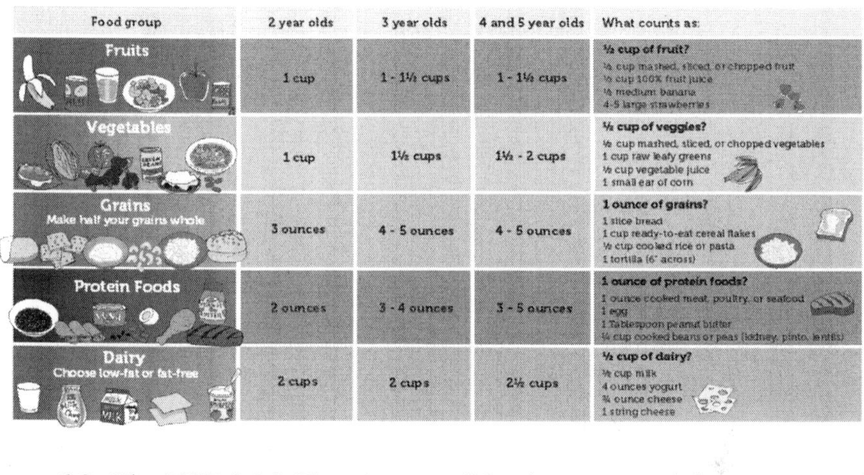

Food group	2 year olds	3 year olds	4 and 5 year olds	What counts as:
Fruits	1 cup	1 - 1½ cups	1 - 1½ cups	**½ cup of fruit?** ½ cup mashed, sliced, or chopped fruit ½ cup 100% fruit juice ½ medium banana 4-5 large strawberries
Vegetables	1 cup	1½ cups	1½ - 2 cups	**½ cup of veggies?** ½ cup mashed, sliced, or chopped vegetables 1 cup raw leafy greens ½ cup vegetable juice 1 small ear of corn
Grains Make half your grains whole	3 ounces	4 - 5 ounces	4 - 5 ounces	**1 ounce of grains?** 1 slice bread 1 cup ready-to-eat cereal flakes ½ cup cooked rice or pasta 1 tortilla (6" across)
Protein Foods	2 ounces	3 - 4 ounces	3 - 5 ounces	**1 ounce of protein foods?** 1 ounce cooked meat, poultry, or seafood 1 egg 1 Tablespoon peanut butter ¼ cup cooked beans or peas (kidney, pinto, lentils)
Dairy Choose low-fat or fat-free	2 cups	2 cups	2½ cups	**½ cup of dairy?** ½ cup milk 4 ounces yogurt ¾ ounce cheese 1 string cheese

Figure 6.3: The USDA MyPlate layout of food groups and the recommended options for each category.

The USDA has formed partnerships with a variety of groups that help endorse MyPlate's messages and reach as many people as possible. These partners are companies/organizations with a national size and scope that have consented to "endorse nutrition content throughout the Dietary Guidelines for Americans." These businesses must adhere to the CNPP's mission and take part in sessions focusing on nutritional design approaches. Numerous national partners, including grocery retailers, health insurers, and food chains support the US Department of Agriculture. MyPlate was hailed as a step forward from the previous MyPyramid logo, which had been critiqued for being too abstract and puzzling (Khorram & Ramezanian, 2021). The 50 percent focus on fruits and vegetables, and also the plate image's simplicity and comprehensibility, were lauded. Because many people struggled to incorporate the Food Pyramid into their daily lives, it was a poor guideline. The general public was confused because many details, such as the suggested daily intake, were left out of this nutritional guideline. MyPlate was the updated version, which included a graphic that made the suggestions very clear and simple to comprehend.

Despite the fact that MyPlate implements nutritionally beneficial dietary guidelines, it does have some drawbacks. The guidelines don't specify plate size, offer snack suggestions, or provide instances of healthy foods for each classification.

Some critics argue that the protein section is superfluous because protein can be found in other food groups and Americans consume enough protein on average; even so, meat does not fit into any of the other food groups. Some people thought the dairy segment was also unnecessary. Another criticism was that the icon is too simple, missing out on chances for additional dietary recommendations, like contrasts between healthy and unhealthy proteins or information on good and bad fats.

In response, the Harvard School of Public Health (HSPH) published the Harvard Healthy Eating Pyramid, an updated and more detailed version of MyPlate. The Healthy Eating Pyramid was proposed as a more up-to-date scientific nutritional findings alternative to MyPlate. Harvard's plate has a higher ratio of vegetables to fruits, includes healthy oils in the recommendation, and divides the plate into equal quarters for healthy (type of) protein and whole grains, as well as recommending water and limiting dairy consumption. "Admittedly, like the previous U.S. Department of Agriculture pyramids, MyPlate mixes science with the impact of influential agricultural interests, which is not the remedy for healthy eating," said Walter Willett, HSPH Chair of the Department of Nutrition (Karthika & Sureshkumar, 2021).

The Harvard plate also includes a physical activity recommendation, which MyPlate frequently overlooks. With an individual's personal weight and exercise routine in mind, these refined dietary regulations state a more accurate methodology to comply with respect to the intake of fats and grains.

The Harvard Medical School also advocates for the incorporation of water in its dietary recommendations.

MyPlate encourages the consumption of milk and other dairy products, but it does not inspire the intake of water. The Healthy Eating Pyramid has a portion on their plate that encourages them to drink more water or non-sugar beverages throughout the day (Jacob *et al.*, 2020).

"There's a huge amount of money at stake in what these regulations say," says Dr. Marion Nestle, former chair of New York University's Department of Nutrition, Food Studies, and Public Health.

"I was told we could never say 'eat less meat' because USDA would not allow it," she said of her work as an HHS and USDA expert.

To Promote Healthy Diets, We Must First Understand Human Nutrition.

Human nutrition is concerned with the supply of essential nutrients in food that are required for human survival and good health. Poor nutrition is a long-term issue that is frequently linked to poverty, food insecurity, or a lack of understanding of nutritional needs (Ibrahim *et al.,* 2015). Malnutrition and its repercussions are major causes of death, physical deformity, and disability all over the world. Nutrition is essential for children's physical and mental growth, as well as for regular human biological development.

Water, carbohydrates, amino acids (found in proteins), fatty acids (discovered in lipids), and nucleic acids are all chemical compounds present in the human body (DNA and RNA). Carbon, hydrogen, oxygen, nitrogen, and phosphorus are all present in these compounds. Any investigation into nutritional status must consider the state of the body beforc and after the experiments, as well as the chemical composition of the entire diet and all substances excreted and eliminated from the body (including urine and feces).

Carbohydrates, fats, fiber, minerals, proteins, vitamins, and water are the seven major types of nutrients. Micronutrients and macronutrients are two types of nutrients (needed in small quantities). Energy is provided by carbohydrates, fats, and proteins, which are macronutrients (Hou & Xu, 2022).

Water and fiber are macronutrients, but they don't contain any energy. Minerals and vitamins are micronutrients.

The macronutrients (except for fiber and water) offer structural and energy content (amino acids, which are used to make proteins, and lipids, which are used to make cell membranes and some activating molecules). Some structural materials can also be used to produce energy internally, and this is recorded in Joules or kilocalories (often referred to as "Calories" and published with a capital 'C' to differentiate them from small 'c' calories).

Carbohydrates and proteins provide 17 kJ (4 kcal) of energy per gram, while fats offer 37 kJ (9 kcal), though the net energy from either is dependent on absorption and digestive effort, which vary widely.

Vitamins, minerals, fiber, and water are not energy-producing substances, but they are necessary for other reasons. Fiber (i.e., non-digestible material like cellulose) appears to be required for complex biochemical purposes, though the actual reason is unknown. Males, on average, need to consume more macronutrients than females across all age groups. In general, until the 2nd or 3rd decade of life, intake levels increase with age (Hathwar *et al*., 2012).

Some nutrients, such as fat-soluble vitamins, can be stored, whereas others are required regularly. An absence of adequate nutrients, and too much of a necessary nutrient in the case of some vitamins and minerals, can lead to poor health. The body cannot synthesize essential nutrients, so they must be obtained from outside sources.

Carbon, hydrogen, and oxygen atoms make up the molecules of carbohydrates and fats. Simple monosaccharides (glucose, fructose, galactose) to complex polysaccharides are all types of carbohydrates (starch). Triglycerides are fatty acid monomers obligated to a glycerol backbone to form fats. Some, but not all, fatty acids are required in the diet because they cannot be produced by the body. In addition to carbon, oxygen, and hydrogen, protein molecules contain nitrogen atoms. Nitrogen-containing amino acids are the building blocks of protein, with some of them being essential because humans cannot produce them on their own (Ferreira & Nunes, 2019). In a process known as gluconeogenesis, some amino acids can be converted to glucose (with the expenditure of energy) and used for energy production just like regular glucose. Internally, some glucose can be produced by breaking down current protein; the residual amino acids are removed, mainly as urea in urine. When atrophy takes place or when a person is starved, this happens naturally.

In the utterances of Marion Nestle, "the list of nutrient content that people are recognized to require is almost certainly incomplete."

6.11 CARBOHYDRATES

Depending on how many monomer (sugar) units they contain, carbohydrates are classified as monosaccharides, disaccharides, or polysaccharides. They're a varied group of chemicals with a variety of chemical, physical, and physiological characteristics. Carbohydrates are found in a variety of foods, including rice, noodles, bread, and other grain-based commodities, but they are not a vital nutrient, meaning that humans do not require them. The brain is the body's largest consumer of sugars, and it consumes a significant amount of glucose, taking into account 20% of total glucose consumption. The brain primarily uses glucose for energy; however, if glucose is insufficient, it switches to fats (Francesconi, 2007).

Monosaccharides have one sugar unit, disaccharides have two sugar units, and polysaccharides have three or more sugar units. Glucose, fructose, and galactose are examples of monosaccharides. Sucrose, lactose, and maltose are disaccharides; purified sucrose, for example, is used as table sugar. Polysaccharides, such as starch and glycogen, are referred to as 'complex' carbohydrates since they are made up of long, multiple-branched bonds of sugar units.

Simple carbohydrates were once thought to be more quickly absorbed and thus raise blood glucose levels faster than complex carbohydrates. This, even so, is incorrect. Some simple carbohydrates (for example, fructose) have different metabolic pathways (for example, fructolysis) that consequence in only partial catabolism to glucose, whereas many complex carbohydrates are metabolized at the same speed as simple carbohydrates. According to the World Health Organization, added sugars should account for no more than 10% of daily energy intake(Acosta-Estrada *et al.*, 2021).

The absorption of starch, the most prevalent plant carbohydrate nutrient, varies. Rapidly digestible starch, slowly digestible starch, and resistant starch are the three types of starch. Plant starches are difficult to digest (resistant starch), but cooking them in the contact with water breaks down the starch granules and emits the glucose chains, making them more digestible by human digestive enzymes. Food was less processed in the past, and starches were encapsulated within the food matrix, finding it challenging to digest. Carbohydrate consumption has moved from less digestible and resistant starch to much more quickly digestible starch as a result of modern food processing. A traditional African diet, for example, contained 38 grams of resistant starch per day. The consumption of resistant starch in regions with high starch intake levels is approximated to be 30-40 grams per day. In the United States, however, the average intake of resistant starch was approximated to be 4.9 grams per day (range 2.8-7.9 grams per day).

6.12 FAT

A dietary fat molecule is usually made up of several fatty acids (long chains of carbon and hydrogen atoms) bonded to a glycerol. Triglycerides are the most common form (three fatty acids attached to one glycerol backbone). Based on the chemical configuration of the fatty acids involved, fats can be defined as saturated or unsaturated. Saturated fats have all of their carbon atoms bonded to hydrogen atoms in their fatty acid chains, whilst unsaturated fats have some of these carbon atoms double-bonded, resulting in molecules with fewer hydrogen atoms than a saturated fatty acid of the same size. Monounsaturated fats (one double bond) and polyunsaturated fats (two double bonds) are two types of unsaturated fats (many double bonds) (Ambuja & Rajakumar, 2018).

Unsaturated fatty acids are also categorized as omega-3 or omega-6 fatty acids based on the position of the double bond in the fatty acid chain. Trans fats are unsaturated fats with trans-isomer bonds that are uncommon and in foods derived from natural sources. They are generally produced in a manufacturing process known as (partial) hydrogenation. Each gram of fat contains nine kilocalories. Fatty acids like conjugated linoleic acid, catalytic acid, eleostearic acid, and punicic acid are powerful immune modulators in addition to providing energy.

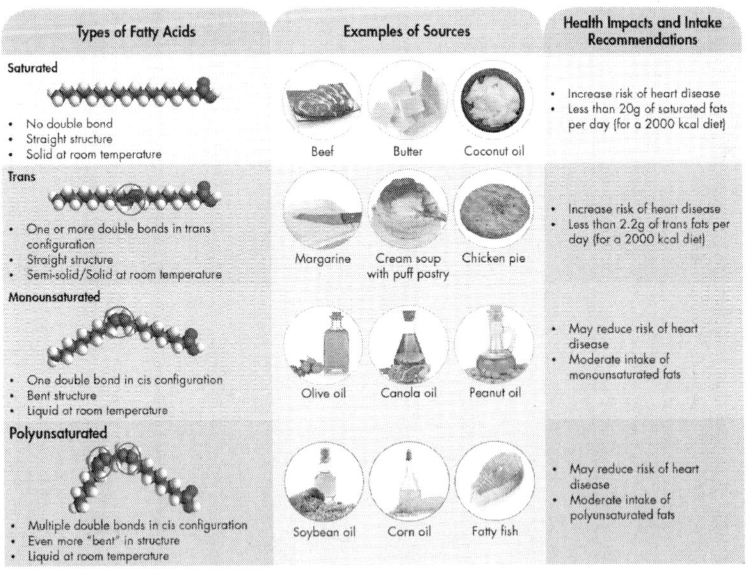

Figure 6.4: Different Types of Dietary Fats and Health.

6.13 FIBER

Dietary fiber is a type of carbohydrate, particularly a polysaccharide, which is poorly absorbed by humans and some animals. When metabolized, it can generate three Calories (kilocalories) of energy per gram, but because of its restricted assimilation and digestibility, it records for less than that in most situations (Yousuf & Siddiqui, 2021).

Dietary fiber can be found in whole grains, beans, and other legumes, fruits (especially plums, prunes, and figs), and vegetables. Bulking, viscosity and fermentation are the three primary mechanisms that determine fiber's health impact. Insoluble fiber helps peristalsis – the rhythmic muscular muscle contraction of the intestines that move substances along the digestive tract – by providing bulk to the intestinal contents. Some soluble and insoluble fibers combine to form a viscous solution, which acts like a gel and slows the passage of food through the intestines (Walker *et al.*, 2015). The microbiome consumes fermentable fibers as food, increasing bulk and generating short-chain fatty acids and other metabolites such as vitamins, hormones, and glucose. Butyrate, one of those other metabolites, is an essential source of energy for colon cells and may help with metabolic syndrome.

6.14 AMINO ACIDS

Proteins are the building blocks of many animal body structures (such as muscles, skin, and hair), as well as the enzymes that regulate chemical reactions in the body. Amino acids, which contain nitrogen and occasionally sulfur, make up each protein molecule. Amino acids are required by the body for the production of new proteins (protein retention) and the replacement of damaged proteins (maintenance). Amino acids are soluble in digestive juices and are absorbed into the blood through the small intestine (Vanbergen & Initiative, 2013). They can't be stored in the body once they've been absorbed, so they're either metabolized or excreted in the urine. Proteins are made up of different proportions of amino acids. From a nutritional standpoint, the amino acid composition of proteins is the most essential part and defining characteristic.

Some amino acids are crucial (an animal can't produce them internally, so they must be consumed) and others are non-essential for all animals (the animal can produce them from other nitrogen-containing compounds). The human body contains approximately twenty amino acids, ten of which are essential. Conditionally essential amino acids are those whose synthesis is limited under certain pathophysiological situations, like prematurity in infants or persons in severe catabolic distress.

In some situations, such as during early growth and differentiation, pregnancy, lactation, or injury, a diet rich in amino acids (especially essential amino acids) is especially important (a burn, for instance). A partial protein source lacks one or more vital amino acids, whereas a complete protein source contains all of them. Protein configurations of two partial protein sources (e.g., rice and beans) can be used to make a complete protein source, and distinct cultural cooking traditions are based on these combinations. Complementary protein sources, on the other hand, do not have to be consumed at the same time for the body to use them together. Excess protein amino acids can be broken down into glucose and used as fuel through gluconeogenesis.

6.15 WATER

The body excretes water in a variety of ways, such as urine and feces, sweating, and water vapor in exhaled breath. As a result, adequate rehydration is forced to fix lost fluids.

Early suggestions for the amount of water required for good health recommended that six to eight cups of water per day was the bare minimum for proper hydration. However, there is no credible scientific source for the claim that a person should drink eight glasses of water per day.

Food-based dietary recommendations:

Water dietary reference values or sufficient daily intakes (ADI). Calculating sufficient intakes from evaluated intakes in populations of people with "desirable osmolarity qualities of urine and attractive water quantities per energy unit consumed" provides these specifications.

The existing EFSA guidelines recommend a total water intake of 2.5 liters per day for healthy hydration. Water from drinking water, other refreshments, and food are included in these reference values. We get about 80% of our water needs from the beverages we consume, with the residual 20% coming from food (Tang et al., 2020). The amount of water in food varies based on the sort of food consumed; for instance, fruit and vegetables contain more water than cereals. These figures are based on food balance sheets for each country published by the Food and Agriculture Organization of the United Nations.

6.16 MINERALS

Other than the four elements carbon, hydrogen, nitrogen, and oxygen, which are present in nearly all organic molecules, dietary minerals are inorganic chemical elements needed by living organisms. Some act as cofactors, while others function as electrolytes. Because the intent is to simply describe the less common elements in the diet, the term "mineral" is archaic. Some are thicker than the four just referenced, such as metals, which are frequently found in the body as ions (Ballester-Sánchez *et al.,* 2019). Some dietitians recommend getting these from foods that naturally contain them, or at the very least as complex compounds, or even from natural inorganic sources. In the ionic forms encountered in such sources, some are assimilated much more freely. Minerals, on the other hand, are frequently artificially taken with food as supplements; the most well-known is probably iodine, which stops goiter and is found in iodized salt.

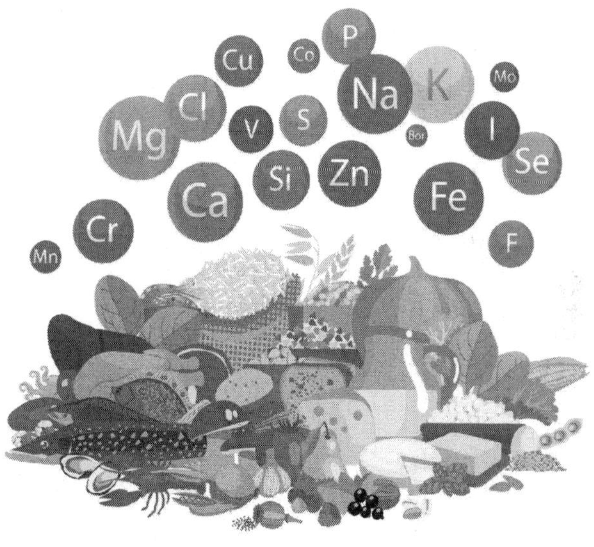

Figure 6.5: Minerals.

6.17 VITAMINS

Vitamins, except vitamin D, are essential nutrients that must be consumed to maintain good health. In the presence of UVB radiation, vitamin D can be synthesized in the skin. (While many animal species can synthesize vitamin C, humans are unable to do so.) Certain vitamin-like compounds, such as carnitine, are thought to be beneficial to survival and health, but they are not "essential" dietary nutrients because the human body can synthesize them from other compounds (Stintzing & Carle, 2004). Furthermore, thousands of distinct phytochemicals have lately been found in food (particularly in fresh vegetables) that may have beneficial properties such as antioxidant activity; however, the experimental demonstration has been inconclusive.

Essential amino acids, essential fatty acids, and the minerals described in the earlier section are examples of essential nutrients that are not classified as vitamins.

Goiter, scurvy, osteoporosis, a weakened immune system, cell metabolism disorders, certain types of cancer, premature aging symptoms, and poor psychological health (such as eating disorders) are just a few of the diseases that vitamin deficiencies can cause.

Excessive amounts of some vitamins can be harmful to one's health. The Institute of Medicine's Food and Nutrition Board has established Tolerable Upper Intake Levels (ULs) for seven vitamins.

CHAPTER 7

CLASSES OF NATURAL PRODUCTS

CONTENTS

Products from plants may be found in a wide range of shapes and sizes. In contrast to the "primary metabolites," which are necessary for plant growth and development, these substances are referred to as "secondary metabolites" instead. In the past, secondary metabolites were seen as "waste products" that had no direct impact on the plant's health. Chemical ecology emerged 30 years ago, and it became clear that these natural products play a significant role in the interactions between plants and their biotic and abiotic environments (Saberi *et al.*, 2017). They may behave as anti-herbivore and anti-pathogen chemicals, pollinator-attracting floral colors, or hormones or signal molecules, for example. Throughout human history, natural products have been employed as food additives, dyes, and pharmaceuticals in addition to their physiological functions in plants.

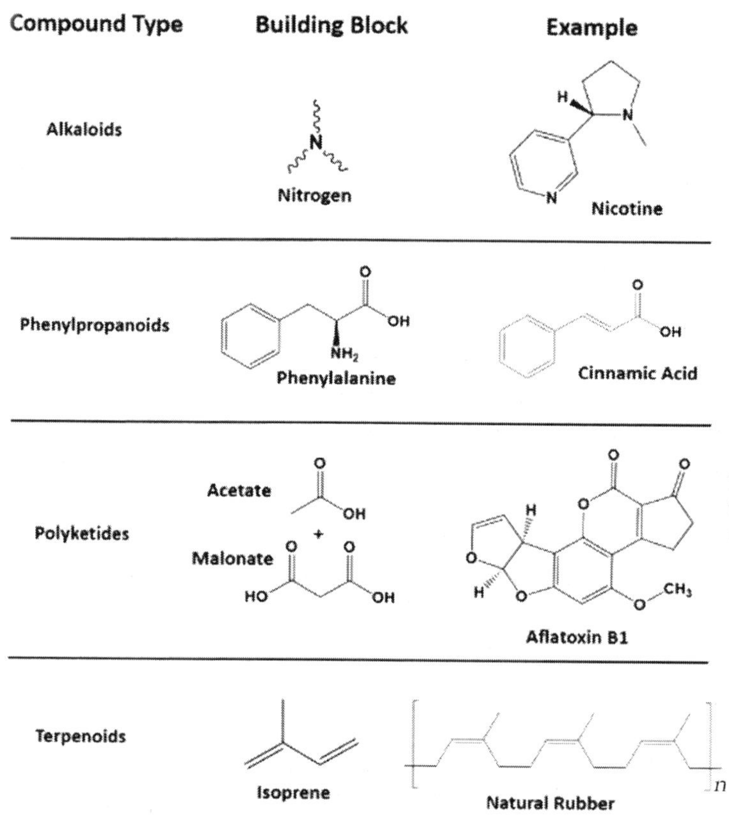

Figure 7.1: Some of the classified elements of natural products.

Humans have been using plants for medicinal, ceremonial, and decorative purposes since time began. Today, there are about 100,000 naturally occurring chemical compounds found in plants, animals, and microorganisms. They are often referred to as natural products, a term that is quite generic. Biomass is the primary source material for bioproducts. As of 2009, biomass accounted for approximately 14% of the global energy supply as well as around 24% of all raw materials used by humans (Dayan *et al.*, 2009).

7.1 CLASSIFICATION OF NATURAL PRODUCTS

There are four major classes of natural products: enzymes, pigments, odors, and toxins. Within these larger classes are many sub-classifications and numerous categories of functional compounds. Also, consist of a large diversity of nonfunctional compounds and non-natural compounds that occur in nature as metabolites. Due to various biological activities, ingestion and application of some natural products have become increasingly important in the field of drug discovery research due to their extraordinary activities in improving human health.

The classification of natural products is divided into primary and secondary metabolites. Secondary metabolites are not essential, they have not been conserved during evolution and are often toxic. They are chemically more complex than primary metabolites and many have only been identified relatively recently. There are several different classes of natural products. Traditionally, they were classified by the mode of occurrence: trace elements, inorganic compounds (minerals), carbohydrates (sugars, polysaccharides), proteins, lipids, and derivatives. Currently, they are most commonly classified according to their biological function and chemical structure: e.g., as a plant-, animal-, or microbial metabolites; as vitamins or coenzymes; and as amino acids, peptides, oligopeptides, polypeptides, polysaccharides (glycans) or oligosaccharides (Rochfort, 2005).

Natural products are also classified into different groups such as herbs and spices, vitamins, essential oils, and minerals. Each grouping is different in the chemical composition, method of preparation and use, medical properties, and specific applications. They are often classified according to their ratio of plant-derived/synthetic ingredients. History has it that even Egyptian kings used natural products in food preparations way back 5000 years ago.

Furthermore, the classification of natural products is the classification of chemicals according to their source. An example of a chemical such as this is caffeine, derived from the coffee plant. This type of categorization can be used to categorize phytochemicals—which include phenols, polyphenols, and terpenes—because they are naturally occurring chemicals in plants.

The eight major classes of natural products include;

- alkaloids,
- phenylpropanoids
- polyketides
- terpenoids
- Tannins
- Saponins
- Steroids
- Flavonoids

7.1.1 Alkaloids

An alkaloid is any of a group of organic nitrogen-containing compounds that contain the basic structural framework necessary to cause an effect on some biological process, examples of which are nicotine in tobacco, and morphine and cocaine in opium poppy. In other words, alkaloids are like "the spice of life", no matter what you're doing or where you're going, you will never be without them! The word alkaloid is derived from the word "alkali". The alkaloids are an amazing, diverse family of organic compounds with numerous functions in living organisms (both plant and animal).

History of alkaloids

Alkaloids are natural products derived from plants, but the word sounds so mysterious that it seems to have come from another world. The history of alkaloids is one of both human ingenuity and resilience. The history of these compounds begins with the first isolation and formation of a pure compound by the Swedish chemist Carl Wilhelm Scheele in 1775 from the leaves of the cinchona tree (Ribeiro et al., 2019). He later named this compound quinine to commemorate its bitter taste. They were then defined in the early 1800s and the term "alkaloid" was coined in 1806. Alkaline substances are always bitter. The first alkaloids were isolated from Solanaceae (nightshade) plants in 1804 by the famous German pharmacist and chemist Feodor Siemens (1792 - 1838).

Alkaloids

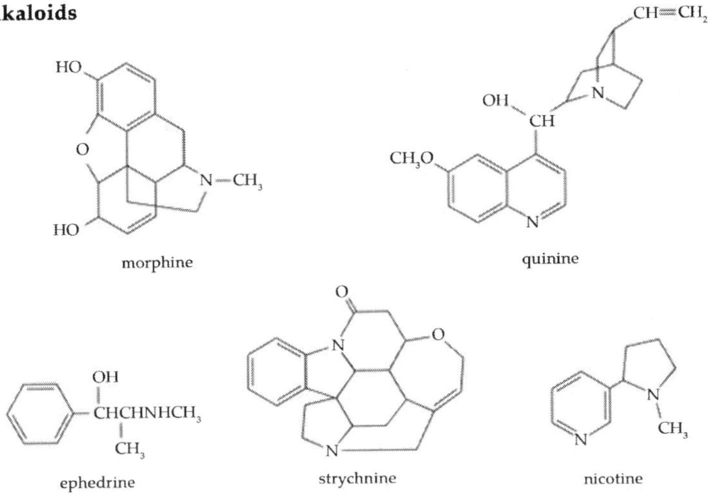

Figure 7.2: The structure of alkaloids.

Hutton was the first to observe that certain plant extracts could interfere with biological systems. In 1864 his discovery of strychnine served as a basis for further investigations on natural products and spurred the development of chemistry research in the late 19th century. The rise of alkaloids and their importance to modern medicine over the last 150 years is at once a history of medicine and a history of chemistry and biology.

Other parties do argue that long ago, a scientist discovered caffeine and was delighted to have found a substance that would help people focus. Later, someone else discovered nicotine and was excited to have found a substance that would help people relax. Unlike the scientist who found caffeine, that person thought nicotine was the only interesting alkaloid... until they discovered psychedelics. In more recent years, scientists have determined that nearly 22% of all pharmaceuticals are derived from plants. The dream of finding nature's remedies was realized by using the highly toxic alkaloids present in plants (Reis *et al*., 2017).

The use of alkaloid compounds as natural products has since grown significantly over the past two decades. This growth is not the result of increased demand for the unique properties these compounds offer, but rather an increased awareness among chemists and biologists that alkaloids can provide solutions to critical challenges faced in a variety of different disciplines. While alkaloids are common in terrestrial organisms, they are not found consistently in all plants as secondary metabolites. Alkaloids are more commonly found in terrestrial organisms than in marine life. However, certain marine organisms such as algae and bacteria synthesize large quantities of highly functionalized alkaloids capable of exhibiting impressive biological activities.

Classification of alkaloids

Alkaloids are a diverse group of naturally-occurring chemical compounds typically found in the plant and semisynthetic drug families. They are considered to be more addictive than cocaine because of the high concentration of serotonin they release when smoked. They are a diverse chemical family in the plant and animal kingdoms, with over seventy thousand members (Raes *et al.*, 2004). They occur widely, particularly in plants and fungi secondary metabolism, as defensive compounds and for the preservation of organisms against the hostility of their external environment.

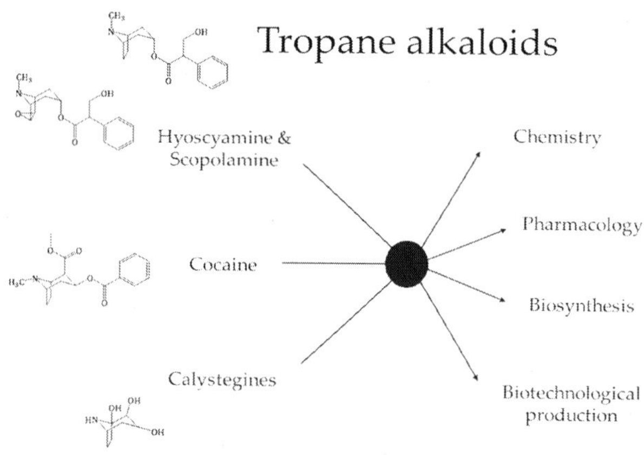

Figure 7.3: Tropane alkaloids are an ester of alkaloids.

Alkaloids can be subdivided by molecular weight, e.g. steroids, tropanes, etc. they are further classified into three distinct groups- nitrogenous, glycosaminoglycan, and cyclic- alkaloids.

Chemistry behind alkaloids

Natural alkaloids are the major structural components of plant and fungal secondary metabolites. They play crucial roles in cell communication. The occurrence of alkaloids is universal and formed by combining nitrogen, carbon, hydrogen, and oxygen atoms in a particular sequence. Some are natural whilst others are synthetic while some can be both (Proksch *et al.*,

2003). These potent little molecules come in a variety of forms: chelating agents, antioxidants, and phytochemistry. Created by plants to help them stay alive, some alkaloids have evolved to become life-saving medicines in humans. They're also responsible for the complex flavors present in tea.

In chemistry, an alkaloid is a heterogeneous group of naturally occurring chemical compounds characterized by a basic nitrogen atom (nitrogenous amine) contained in a ring structure. This group also includes some related compounds with neutral and even weakly acidic properties. Some synthetic derivatives of additional nitrogen-containing compounds, such as caffeine, are also termed alkaloids. The more extended definition of Alkaloids includes the morphinan and steroid class of plant compounds. Alkaloids are natural products derived from plants, animals, and bacteria that may have physiological actions on humans. Many alkaloids with important medicinal properties occur as secondary metabolites in plants, particularly in the sap (extracts) and leaves (Pop. *et al.*, 2019).

There are different chemical structures and organic frameworks that alkaloids can form i.e. 1. stereoisomer 2. Tautomerism. Alkaloids contain at least one basic (alkaline) hydrogen ion, or proton and which can form stable salts with various metal ions. Many alkaloids also contain sulfur and are therefore called hydrates. They can be derived from the following classes of animals: Opisthokonta, Rhizopoda, Porifera, Coelenterata, Echinodermata, Brachiopoda, Annelida, Arthropoda, and Mollusca.

It was Wernicke who discovered that, when mixed with water, some alkaloids dissolved in a ring. Sounded like part of a wedding ceremony. He called these ringed compounds "a-pyridines." This Greek-sounding name came from the fact that the same compounds had been previously isolated and named by E. Merck. He named them "phenizins," which is a Greek word meaning, "to give off smoke/smell," referring to their unpleasant odor/ taste.

Effects of alkaloids on plants and animals

Alkaloids are bitter and have physiological effects on humans including, antiseptics, stimulants, hallucinogenic, and cancerous agents. They have the distinction of being able to produce an effect on human beings; indeed some alkaloids are medicinally active, though most are not. Alkaloids are not that bad to be around. In plants, they can help the plant absorb calcium and phosphorus. While this might explain some interesting side effects in sheep and cattle, it doesn't seem to have much of an effect on humans.

Alkaloids are chemicals that occur naturally in vascular plants and animals. These chemicals affect organisms in several different ways; they can be used as a protection mechanism or as a defense mechanism by the plant or animals. When ingested they can cause harm to the predator or herbivore who has eaten the food source. Alkaloids can also be used in medicine for inflammation, proteins, and RNA and DNA synthesis (Da Silva *et al.*, 2016). The active compounds in both plants and animals are called alkaloids. Organic chemists investigate the structures and reactions of alkaloids to better understand the mechanisms with which organisms synthesize them. Their findings illuminate strategies by which a cell produces any kind of chemical compound. Some alkaloids have been shown to have favorable effects concerning crop height and weight, bio-immunostimulation, disease resistance, stress resistance, etc. It is hypothesized that the favorable effect of alkaloids on plants is due to their ability to scavenge the oxygen radicals and thereby restore the physiological activity of crops. The alkaloids contained within a plant are produced by the plant itself, forming a complex defense system against predators. Left-over alkaloids are bad tasting and often poisonous to animals.

7.1.2 Phenylpropanoids

Phenylpropanoids are molecules that are chemically close to citric acid and salicylic acid, as well as some other closely related compounds. The first part of their name is phenyl, which is a chemical group containing a benzene ring and two adjacent hydroxyl groups. They play many roles in biological processes, such as the biosynthesis of lignin and quinoids. It is a category of around 300 small molecules which are formed as intermediate products in the synthesis of various phenolic compounds. Phenylpropanoids are formed by the phenylpropanoids, derived from 3-Phosphoglycerate (3-PGA), which can be found ubiquitously in plants and also in animals.

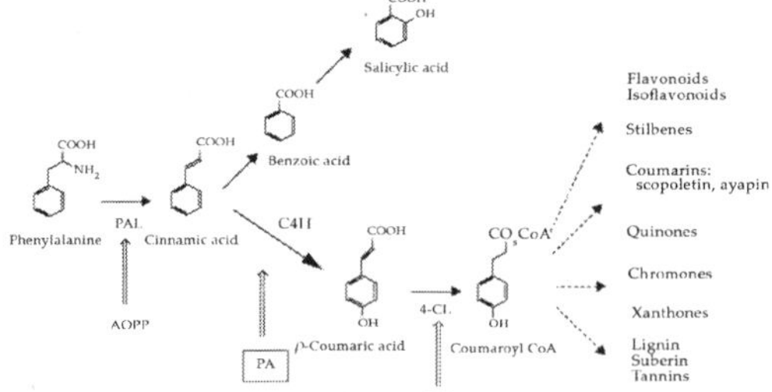

Figure 7.4: The structure of phenylpropanoid.

They are also called phenolic acids. They are further biosynthesized by phenylalanine ammonia-lyases (PALs) in plants and fungi. The genes encoding the PAL enzymes that produce phenylpropanoids have been identified in many plant species. Closely related to phytohormones, phenylpropanoids are present in a wide variety of plants and play an important role in many biological processes (Odhaib *et al.*, 2021). In this case, phenylpropanoid nomenclature refers, however, not to the complex breakdown products of auxin, but rather to the simple phenols that can be isolated from plant laticiferous tissue using basic techniques. Members of this class have diverse biological functions and can be found in all kingdoms of life

History of phenylpropanoids

Phenylpropanoids were first isolated from propolis over 100 years ago, as reported by Auguste Cahours in 1899. Still today, these wonderful phenylpropanoids are derived from propolis because of their health-promoting attributes. Much to the surprise of several scientists, the history of phenylpropanoids begins with two products that are more commonly categorized as ketones - quinoid and purine. In the beginning, they were likely just curious substances associated with folklore medicine, but once science came along, they became tools to discover and develop new interesting things.

In part, research into this folklore medicine was prompted by the early work of Louis Pasteur while he was pioneering studies into fermentation, which led him to believe that certain naturally occurring chemicals called phenylpropanoids were responsible for a plant's capacity to affect fermentation. Phenylpropanoids are a diverse family of plant products that have been the subject of intense research for decades. They are naturally occurring, perhaps rather highly underrated, small molecules that can be found at numerous sites in the plant kingdom, but most abundantly in the bark and wood of conifers (Murdoch *et al.*, 2000). In more recent years, phenylpropanoids have also been found in leaves, flowers, and fruits, as well as in fungi and microorganisms. However, and unfortunately, not all phenylpropanoid-containing plants produce large amounts of phenylpropanoids. Thus, when analyzing the history of phenylpropanoids one can say that it is a long and winding story also because many of the key plant species (meta phenylene) occur sporadically and consequently are difficult to find.

Chemistry behind phenylpropanoids

Phenylpropanoids are biosynthesized from the transformation of shikimic acid by an array of enzymatic reactions catalyzed by phenylalanine ammonia-lyase (PAL), amino acid decarboxylases, hydroxycinnamoyl transferases (HCT), hydroxycinnamoyl CoA ligases (HCCL), aromatic hydroxylase and dihydroflavonol reductase (DFR). This compound consists of a benzene ring replaced by a propane chain. The term is also applied to the corresponding class of chemical compounds, the phenylpropanoids. The phenylpropane structure is an intermediate between the aromaticity of benzene and the alkane structure of propane.

Chemical and biological studies of phenylpropanoid metabolism in plants have received major attention in recent decades due to the role of these compounds in agriculture, medicine, and daily life. Phenylpropanoids are used as plant growth hormones and play a vital role in both plant physiology and molecular genetics. The Phenylpropanoids include some biologically active compounds with the most familiar being tannins and lignans. These compounds are present in plants, especially those serving to prevent infection or acting as chemical defense systems. Recent work has brought some of these compounds and the processes by which they are synthesized, into the spotlight and represents what is considered to be an interesting biochemical window into evolution (Multari *et al*., 2015).

A major component of the chemical structure of flavonoids, phenylpropanoids are naturally occurring compounds that give oils their color and organic flavors. They are also responsible for the browning of fruits exposed to air. In addition to health-promoting actions, phenylpropanoids can promote several technological applications such as extraction and purification of oil, production of vitamin C and enzymes, pesticides, flavorings and fragrances, dyes, and pigments.

Phenylpropanoids are multifunctional molecules involved in the metabolism of a large number of plant species. The phenylpropanoids play a crucial role in the life cycle of plants. Their key metabolites are involved in plant defense, plant structure and metabolism, cellular functions and regulation, environmental interactions, and signaling cascades. Phenylpropanoid biosynthesis is a highly regulated process that allows the plant to adapt to environmental conditions, survive environmental stresses, and prevent disease. They are frequently associated with plants' defense mechanisms against feeding insects and other herbivores. They play a critical role in biochemical processes such as pollination and seed formation, making them critical to many agroforestry systems. Phenylpropanoids also serve as precursors to various drug compounds that have been shown to modulate various physiological processes in humans and animals.

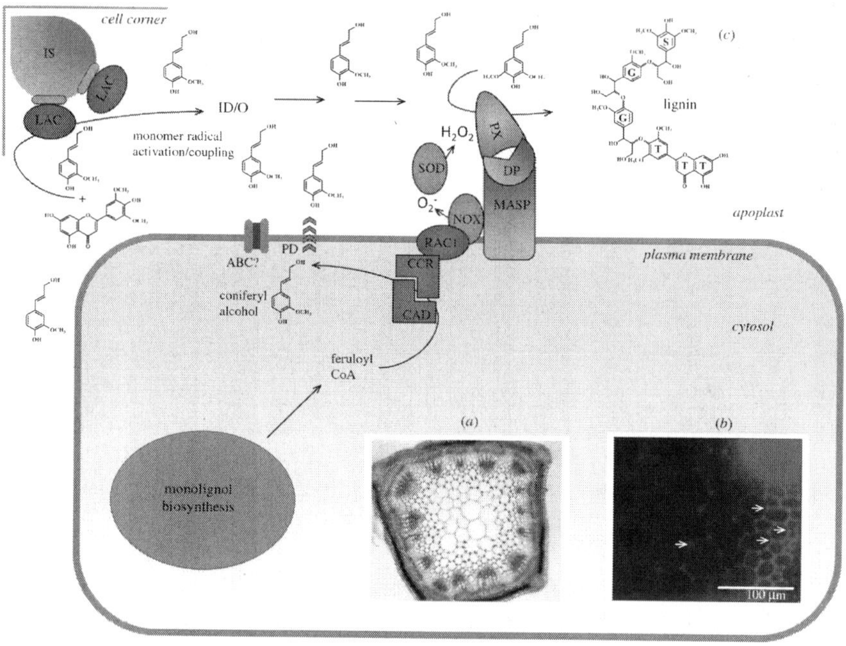

Figure 7.5: Initiation of lignification which represents the UV protection through lignin and flavonoid accumulation in plant cell.

They combine the structures of phenols and a hindered propane-2-one group. They belong to the group of phytohormones, more known as brassinosteroids, which bind to specific receptors inside their target cells. The DNA of each species is similar in structure and sequence to that of others, with about 98% similarity between humans and rice for example. Some slight variations in nucleotide sequence can alter gene expression or produce a frameshift mutation that causes deletions, additions, or substitutions in the amino acid sequence of the final protein (Lin et al., 2010). Nuclear genetic mutations may be inherited from parents and passed on to offspring. These variations appear in populations naturally through random changes or mutations during DNA replication and are referred to as polymorphisms. Perhaps the most important advances have concerned better methods of plants for disease control, pesticides for insecticides against insect pests, and newer techniques for enhancing products such as biofuel production and silviculture.

Functions of phenylpropanoids

Also known as phenolics, they are synthesized by plants for a range of functions, including UV protection through lignin and flavonoid accumulation in plant cell walls and repelling predators through the production of tannins. They play important roles in plant growth, reproduction, and defense against insects.

Phenylpropanoids are the major constituents of lignins, which are building blocks of vascular plants. Lignins are synthesized via the phenylpropanoid pathway and their functions include structural components of plant cell walls, pigments, and lignin derivatives. They have also been shown to have the potential of acting as antioxidants, anticancer, anti-inflammatory, antitumor agents, etc (Linares *et al.,* 2017). In particular, flavonoids constitute a major class of phenolic secondary metabolites in living organisms. It is well documented that phenolic compounds modulate various physiological activities by regulating the degree of pro-oxidant/antioxidant activities or influence both cellular and organism responses to therapy.

Examples of phenylpropanoids

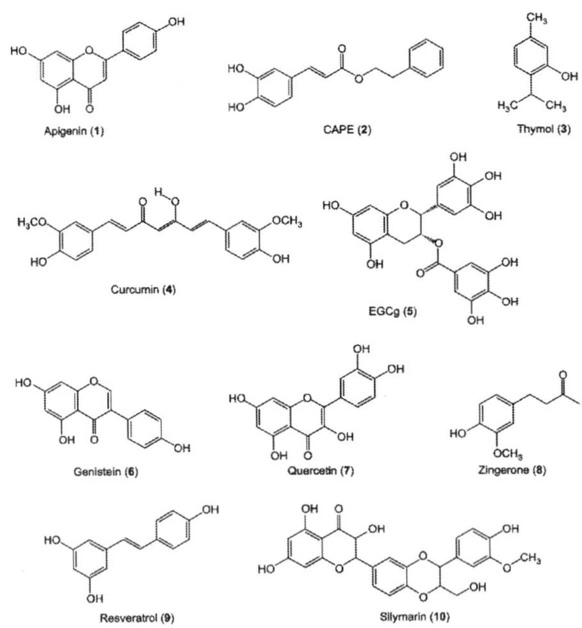

Figure 7.6: A sample example of phenylpropanoids.

Phenylpropanoids are a diverse family of natural compounds derived from phenylalanine and derived from this. Due to the close connection between phenylpropanoid metabolism and the biosynthesis of secondary metabolites, their diversity is even wider. They represent a large family of metabolites that have been reported in about 20,000 species belonging to all major divisions of the plant kingdom: angiosperms, gymnosperms, ferns, and mosses. These derivatives of the shikimic acid-derived benzoic acid are found among as many as 400 plant species, including cranberries. Examples of phenylpropanoids include salicin, tannins, resveratrol, and phytophenols.

7.1.3 Polyketides

Polyketides, also called macrolides, are a group of large biological molecules. Polyketides are a very diverse group of compounds encompassing a broad range of natural products including antibiotics like erythromycin and vancomycin. They represent a class of naturally occurring polyketides found in fungi. Polyketides are essential to the field of natural product chemistry (López *et al*., 2019). They are formed by the large-scale condensation of multiple acetate carbons in a repeating isoprenoid unit. The enzymes involved in the biotic and abiotic synthesis of these compounds have become attractive targets for drug discovery. Furthermore, are a heterogeneous and structurally diverse class of macrolide antibiotics of various classes (antibacterials and antitubercular), but also include immunosuppressants and even anticancer agents.

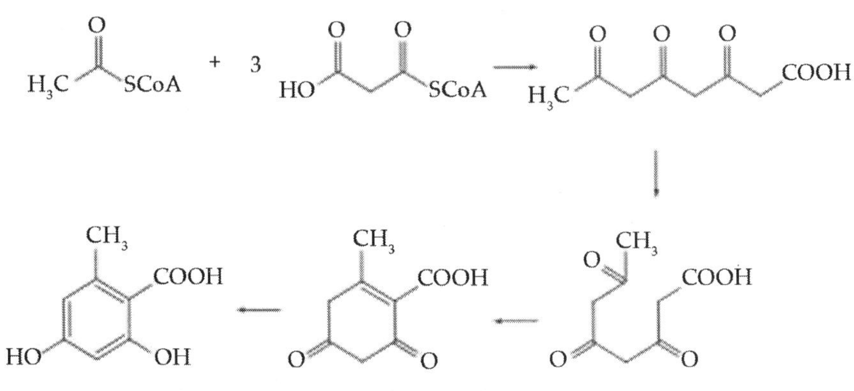

Figure 7.7: The structure of polyketide.

Polyketides comprise a large and important class of natural products that include many clinically significant antibiotics. Polyketides play important roles in quinone-mediated redox and many of the polyketide metabolites have been found to have pharmacological activities. The most well-known members include tetracyclines, macrolides, phthalides, and mangoes. Many polyketides are cytotoxic and are known to target numerous microorganisms including *Escherichia coli*, *Encephalitozoon cuniculi*, *Histoplasma capsulatum*, *Streptococcus pneumoniae*, *Cryptococcus neoformans*, *Plasmodium falciparum*, Malaria parasite protozoan, intracellular parasite Apicomplexa, extracellular parasite *Trypanosoma brucei* (Trypanosomatidae), *Bacteroides fragilis* (Bacteroidaceae) and *Mycobacterium tuberculosis* (Karioti *et al.*, 2015).

History of polyketides

Polyketides have been regarded as the top ten greatest discoveries in Natural Product Chemistry by C&EN, the American Chemical Society. A collection of papers trace the development of polyketide research from the early days when its chemistry was considered unsophisticated, to the current status as a burgeoning medicinal field. Coverage includes biosynthesis, industrial applications, biotechnology, and pharmacology.

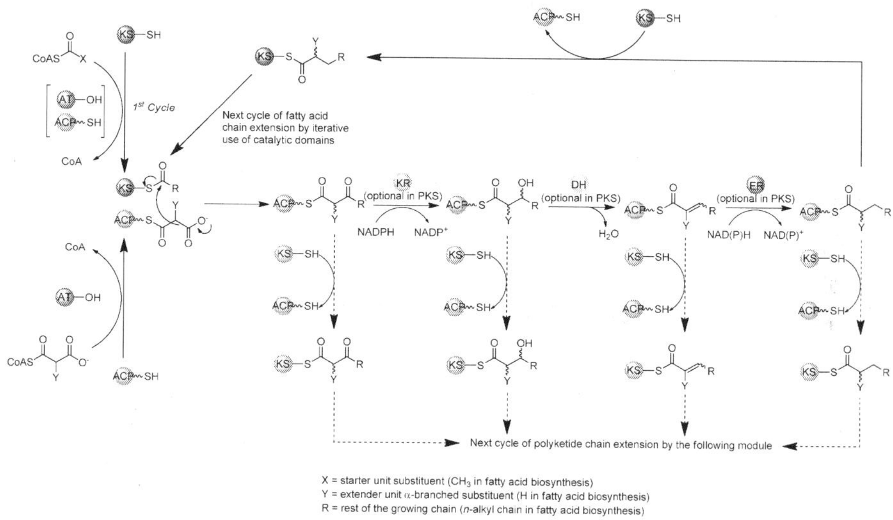

Figure 7.8: The biosynthesis of polyketides.

(Source: Kwan DH, and Schulz F.,2011)

The history of polyketides is traced from the discovery of vinblastine in *Vinca rosea* in 1820, along with two other alkaloids, to a more complete understanding of their biosynthesis. The development of techniques for investigating and synthesizing natural products, the elucidation of secondary metabolite pathways, and the role played by biotechnology in discovering new metabolites have expanded over time.

Based on the carbon skeletons of mevalonic acids, they contain more than 15000 members from 800 genera and 45 families, which are produced by bacteria, fungi, and plants recent studies have highlighted the interesting historical developments of polyketides in both plants and microbes. Plant polyketides were first discovered by Hinman in 1876 as pigments extracted from plants. Many compounds of plant origin have been studied historically or are still being investigated in the present day (Dixon & Sumner, 2003).

Within the last decade, next-generation sequencing technologies have uncovered vast new resources of genetic information that have not been available previously to scientists and have opened a new era in genome research with the discovery of multiple non-ribosomal peptide synthetases (NRPSs) and polyketide synthases (PKSs) genes. Today, polyketides play prominent roles in contemporary biomedical research. For example, they have led to the most widely used class of antibiotics, are responsible for the red color of some toxins produced by dinoflagellates, and they often attract great attention in drug discovery programs.

Chemistry behind polyketides

Polyketides are secondary metabolites, that is, they are synthesized along a biochemical pathway unrelated to primary metabolism. Production of polyketides occurs mainly in the cytosol and plastids of micro-organisms. There are two major types: i) linear polyketides (L-type) and ii) cyclic polyketides (C-type). The structures of various polyketides consist of substituted phenyl or heterocyclic rings with an alkyl side chain connected to the terminal carbon atom by a thioacetal bond. A polyketide is a kind of natural product molecule produced by the assembly of ketides by enzymes called polyketide synthases (Khorram & Ramezanian, 2021).

Its backbone consists of five or six carbons (five-membered and six-membered lactone rings). They are synthesized via polyketide synthase enzymes and typically contain an N-acetylglucosaminyl residue at their branch points. Polyketides are produced by nonribosomal peptide synthetases (NRPS). Many of these enzymes are encoded by modular multienzyme complexes called polyketide synthases (PKSs) or hybrid PKS/NRPS systems.

The polyketide synthases responsible for the synthesis of this group of important natural products have been studied extensively in bacteria and fungi, as well as in the plant and animal kingdoms. Polyketides represent a large family of linear or branched polymers of carbon subunits, that are composed of carbonyl groups (C=O) joined by carbon-carbon bonds.

In the laboratories, this natural product is reproduced by the assembly of monomer molecules into longer chain molecules using enzymes encoded by type I and type II polyketide synthase genes (PKS genes). Many important biomedicines and natural products containing drugs are produced by this mechanism, which is similar to fatty acid biosynthesis (Fabani *et al.*, 2013).

Functions of polyketides

Ough polyketides are most commonly known in nature as antibiotics and other pharmaceuticals, they also play a significant role in as many as 80% of plants. Some are co-opted for use by humans—for example, the pharmaceutical reserpine is derived from the roots of an Indian medicinal plant. Indeed, most products from polyketides have therapeutic activity. They include drugs such as statins and taxol, compounds used to treat cardiovascular disease and cancer. They are also used as antibiotics and immunosuppressants. Although not produced by bacteria or fungi, they are involved in the signaling pathways of both groups. Polyketide natural products have been proven to have antimicrobial properties, anti-tumor, and anti-inflammatory properties, thus showing great potential for clinical use.

Examples of polyketides

Polyketides are natural polymers (carbohydrates) that have in common a poly-β-keto backbone. For example, the polyketide backbone of resveratrol is shown on the left. Polyketides often are aromatic and can be important as antibiotics or pigments. Lately, synthetic biologists have developed an interest in these compounds because of their commercial value and the complexity of their assembly pathways (Karthika & Sureshkumar, 2021). Examples of polyketides are daphnetin, saxitoxin, applying B, and hypotaurine. Furthermore, they are generally defined as a group of antibiotics such as streptomycin, tetracycline, erythromycin, macrolide, and taxol.

Synthons are hypothetical intermediates of polyketide biosynthesis. They are characterized by the removal of the homologous containing nucleophilic functions to be able to undergo the retro-Claisen condensation so that the C (14)=C(15) double bond is established.

7.1.4 Terpenoids

Terpenoids are a natural product that is derived from pine resin and contains tar and terpenes originating from pine which has been shown to have powerful anti-inflammatory properties and aromatherapy benefits. It is the next-generation fungicide containing purified metabolites, an entirely botanical polymer mix, and a patented complex of actives. The product has been specifically formulated to kill the tar spot fungus and its spores while protecting the most vulnerable part of the plant. It is completely safe for use on roadside trees, shrubs, flowers, vegetables, fruits, and turf. Terpenoids are available in a ready-to-use spray bottle or in a concentrated concentrate to be diluted before application.

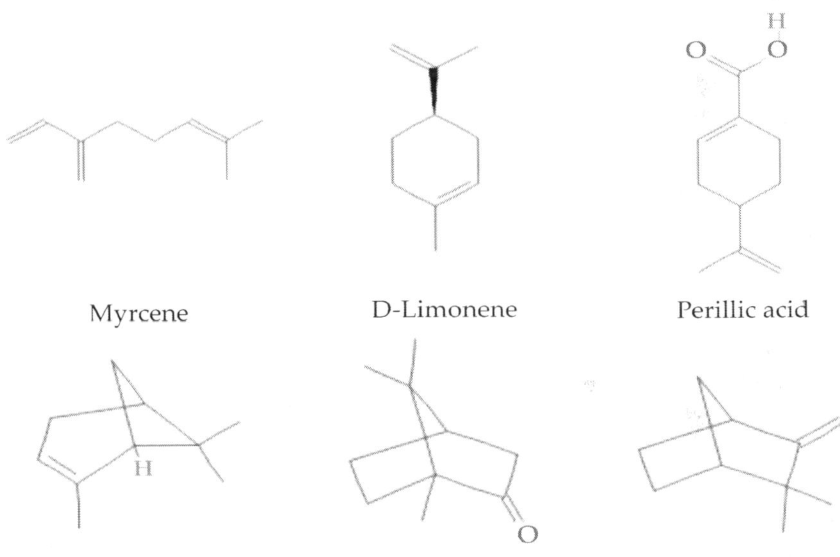

Figure 7.9: The structure of terpenoid.

(Source: Proshkina E, Plyusnin S, et al.,2020)

Other definitions argue terpenoids are a natural product using the oils of pine tar, a renewable resource and natural biodegradable solvent for a safer environment. Terpenoids are mixed with petroleum distillate to produce an effective, environmentally safe cleaning solution that is great for removing wax build-up, paint and clear coats, rail dust, salt deposits from winter road salts, and much more. The term "tar" is derived from the Latin word "turpentinus", meaning "of the turpentine tree".

Frankly, terpenoids represent a collection of natural products. The collection includes all the carrier oils, kinds of butter, and waxes that we believe you'll need to create sensational and efficacious products. Whether you are looking to make exquisite massage oil or a luxurious hand cream. Terpenoids have the right ingredients to allow you to create exceptional products (Karwowska *et al.,* 2021).

History of terpenoids

The history of Terpenoids is a fascinating one, with discoveries made over 150 years ago still relevant in today's scientific world. It begins with an extract from a resin found in the Middle East. Used as a medicinal remedy for thousands of years, this extract was highly prized by those who traveled across the desert. With the decline of the Ottoman Empire in the early 20th century, this valuable secret was lost. In the 1930s, a chemist from The University of Minnesota developed a formula to replicate the natural resin and create a terpenoid product.

However, some people believe that terpenoids were first discovered in Tarpeny. The historians argue that the discovery was near the city of Tarpeny, a tiny town near the Italian border. This Italian-based organic compound was first introduced to industrialists in 1872. It is said Terpenoids played a valuable role in the development of modern plastics, paints, and pharmaceuticals.

The powerful organic compounds are now produced widely around the world and have become a key component in many organic products and cosmetics such as makeup and shampoos (Francesconi, 2007).

These terpenoids have been used in Japan and China as potent biocides for a long time. Having a very high molecular mass and exhibiting multiple positive charges, they cannot be broken down easily by conventional techniques of removing foreign microbes from water. The particular history of terpenoids is rooted in the ancient days when sailors and pirates often suffered from an ailment referred to as scurvy.

This disease affected their ability to perform as a result of their diets lacking sufficient vitamin C. In 1817, with the completion of HMS Brazen, the issue was realized and research began. The conclusion yielded 3 sources: lemons, burnets, and oranges. This special mixture contained oranges, lemon juice, sugar, and unrefined spirits, which resulted in scurvy resistance.

Chemistry and biosynthesis behind terpenoids

The Terpenoids product is derived from the leaves of a pine tree. These leaves possess a substance called terpene that is extracted and mixed with other ingredients including alcohol to create a natural oil product. The pine bark is extracted and then boiled down to produce oil which is then turned into various products. It can also be derived from nontreated Arabica coffee beans. This natural material can inhibit the growth of molds and fungi on materials.

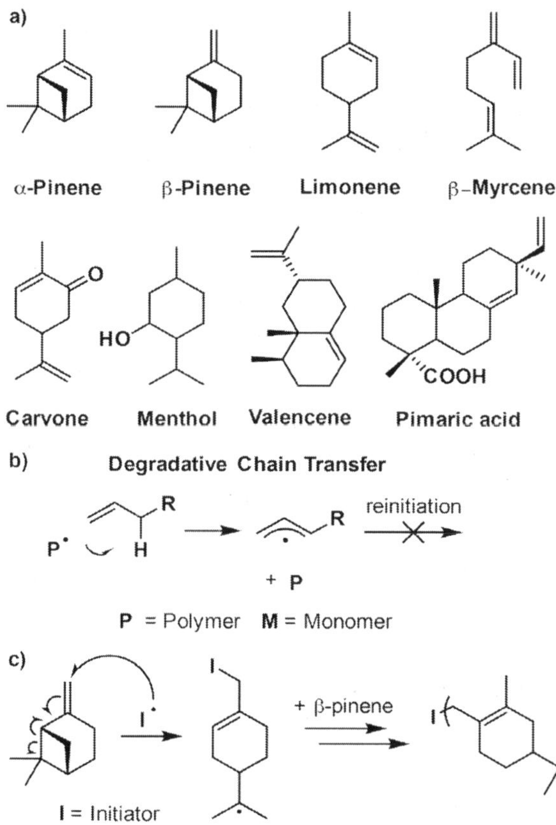

Figure 7.10: A selection of naturally occurring terpenoids.

Terpenoids and fluorinated natural products are the latest class of compounds to emerge from isoprene and the most complex naturally occurring molecules. Terpenoids do not contain any dangerous and potentially harmful chemicals. Terpenoid, a bicyclo [3.3.0] octane ring system with a trans-4,4′-dimethyl configuration at the bridgehead positions, is one of the most common carbon skeletons found in natural products. An understanding of the chemistry of this class of compounds is important because they are so common in nature and because they represent a significant class of drugs and other biologically active molecules.

This aromatic compound consists of a nucleobase, 1 or more sugar moieties and at least one phosphate group, they also contain additional chemical elements such as sodium, potassium, zinc, and magnesium. The bio-synthetic origin and diversity of Terpenoids have been a breakthrough with the synthesis of the skeleton of terpenoids. It can be used by using the organic polymer as a protective covering (Kau et al., 2011). They are found in phospholipids which are a major component in cell membranes. This Diversity exists in thousands of different forms.

Functions of terpenoids

Actively inhibits disease progression at the cell wall level allowing nutrients to enter plants. Multi-site of action and easy to use, expands the choice growers have in their disease management program against a wide range of pathogens including Botrytis, Sclerotinia, Alternaria, Fusarium, and Sulfur fungus. Terpenoids are also used for repelling mosquitoes, flies, and other pests that can spread disease. It is the only product with two federally registered uses: a fertilizer and an insecticide. It has the added advantage of being slow-release, so the dosages are small.

This natural product is also effective against the most common parasites of lawns, ornamentals, and crops. Common parasite species include white grubs, chinch bugs, billbugs, and sod webworms. Terpenoids are further powerful, concentrated cleaners for sparkling results on all surfaces. Because Terpenoids with their plant-based ingredients come from nature, one doesn't need to worry about using them near food or in the kitchen (Ferreira & Nunes, 2019).

Terpenoids further help people with heavy periods, menorrhagia, bad cramps, and nausea with their monthly menstrual cycle. The natural product is rich in polyphenols that achieve instant color intensification and long-term clarity.

7.1.5 Tannins

Tannin is a natural product derived from the bark of grapevines. These powerful antioxidants have been shown to improve cardiovascular and circulatory health, as well as support healthy skin, hair, and eyes. It is formulated with

8 ingredients, including tannic acid from seed husks of organically grown Barberry fruit. They are also made from pure Mediterranean grape seeds rich in antioxidants and flavonoids and are ideal for adding flavor to animal proteins like beef, pork, chicken, lamb and seafood. They are also derived from tree bark. In addition to this, tannins are extracted during the process of producing tea leaves. Tannins will prevent the breakdown of the tannins, preserving the original color, taste, and nutrients. It binds the color to pure cellulose fibers or leather. It is completely water-soluble but will retain its effectiveness even after 9 months.

Trees produce tannin to help protect themselves by making their outer bark more resistant to breakage and to reduce bacterial growth. The high tannin content, along with the astringent qualities of tannins help control erosion, stabilize soil and nutrients, increase water retention and improve soil aeration. They can also be defined as a group of compounds that bind to proteins, starches, and carbohydrates to help impart the astringent mouth feel found in red wines. Tannins aren't isolated to red wine either, as many plants contain those including raisins, barley, and cocoa.

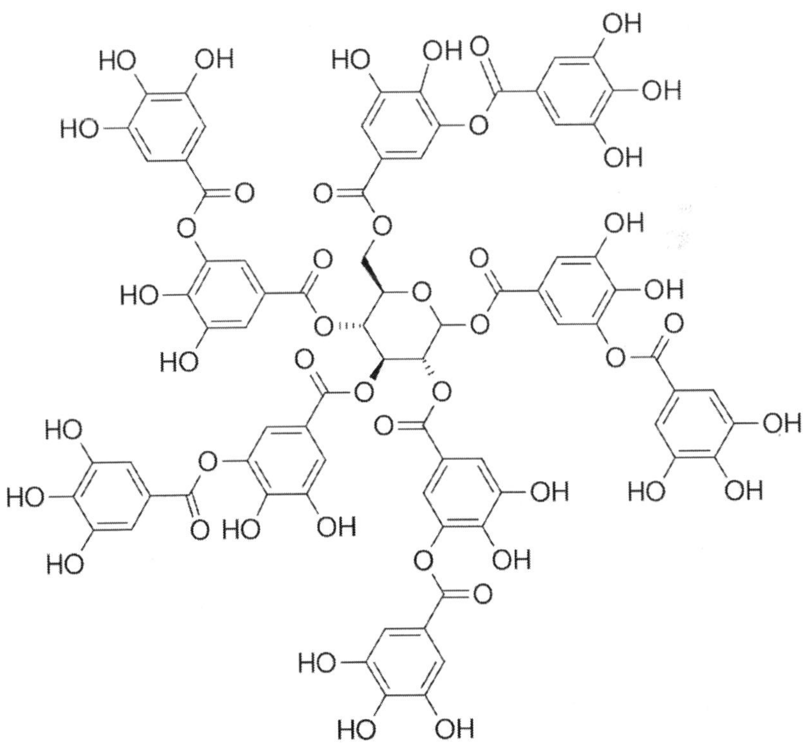

Figure 7.11: The structure of Tannin.

History and diversity of Tannins

The use of tannins in human affairs pre-dates recorded history. Tannins are polyphenolic compounds that have been used for centuries to tan leather hides. They were also used medically (poultices and herbal remedies) in many early cultures. However, it was not until the 1970's that further studies revealed their antioxidant properties and many other beneficial effects in animal feeding trials. Present-day research includes the study of their benefits in healthy foods and supplements, especially for cardiovascular nutrition, anti-inflammatory protocols, antimicrobial results, cancer chemoprotective properties, etc. Tannins have been used since antiquity as dyes, tanning agents, and astringents. Tannins are found in large amounts in the bark of many trees, notably the oak (*Quercus* spp.). Concentrated tannins have also been isolated from the leaves of several plant species, such as *Acacia catechu* (Hathwar *et al*., 2012).

The unique and versatile properties of tannins have been at the heart of medicine, textiles, food and wine technology, animal husbandry, and human nutrition over the centuries. Tannins being used as mordants predate the use of metals. Tanning is believed to have been discovered accidentally during the process of preserving animal hides upon exposure to smoke and sunlight.

Now, due to developments in chemical and analytical methods, it is possible to concentrate on the numerous physiological functions of tannins in plants. There is an enormous number of tannin compounds; many have never been chemically defined and most of them remain unidentified. Investigations on the biosynthesis and occurrence in plants are increasingly providing new insights into the versatile modes of action of tannins as regulators of plant growth and cell function and as defense compounds against pathogens and grazing animals.

The chemistry and bio-synthesis behind tannins

The chemistry and bio-synthesis of Tannins, as a natural product has been the focus of scientific research in the last decade, mainly with emphasis on the enzymatic and chemical reaction involved, as well as its role in wine and other beverages. Tannins appear in many forms and have diverse origins (Halloran et al., 2015). Possible confusion of Tannins with the polymerization products of the amino acid tryptophan and glucose have been removed. The synthesis of Tannins is explained by the reaction between extractives soluble in water and polymerizable tannin precursors insoluble in water.

In recent years, the research area of tannin has been extensively investigated because of the biocompatible property of tannins. The purpose of this book is to provide an up-to-date review of the chemistry and biosynthesis of tannins. What's more, some popular herbs such as *Camellia silences*, *Camellia assamica*, *Cymbopogon citratus,* and others are introduced by their tannin contents. Tannins are the second largest class of polyphenols (phenolic compounds) after flavonoids and display large structural diversity. Their derivates, the mono- and oligosaccharides which are produced upon hydrolysis of tannins are collectively known as pyrogallolpolynucleotides or 'PGN'. The PGNs are mainly derived from Tannin, Galloylglucose (2, 3: 1, 4-Glucan), but also occur in other plant polymeric substances such as inositol and xylose polymers. So far, over 70 individual tannins have been identified in plants and coal tar.

The natural product is common to most vascular plants holding great chemical, biochemical and industrial importance. They serve as phytochemical defense mechanisms against herbivores, fungal infections and senescent or abnormal growth processes. Their abstract synthesis yields products relevant to pharmaceutical research, chemical ecology, and other industrial applications.

Functions of Tannins

Tannins eliminate iron and hydrogen from the water. It helps to prevent stains, especially on tile and grout. It also fights the effects of rosacea. With its soothing and protective qualities, it is one of the very few products on the market formulated for those suffering from this condition. The natural product tannin is also used in the cloth industry. It helps extend the life of clothes. It allows for better water attachment to the fibers, which is why it results in clothing that does not wrinkle as easily and lasts longer (Haque *et al.*, 2020). Tannins also help to reduce and eliminate any odor to your clothes that often comes from washing with soap. They inhibit the growth of mold and yeast, restore luster to faded fabrics and reduce static charge in synthetic fabrics.

Tannin products strengthen and benefit leather and other materials by infusing the skin with their special characteristics to produce a beautiful natural look that improves with age. Just a small amount will infuse the leather with this amazing characteristic. Tannins also help keep fish healthy by removing organic pollutants, such as nitrogen and phosphorous, from pond water. Tannins can be used continuously for one or two weeks at a time with no negative side effects on temperature or oxygen levels. Most importantly, Tannins allow fish to grow up cleanly and strong instead of having to resort to antibiotics.

The natural product is also perfect for both red and white winemaking. It provides a pleasant drying sensation known as "astringency" and helps to round out the mid-palate. This product also helps remove excess protein which may precipitate during bottle aging. These compounds have both positive and negative health effects: they exert antioxidant activity and anti-carcinogenic effects but also interfere with iron absorption (Hou & Xu, 2022).

7.1.6 Saponins

Saponins are natural products that have been used for more than eight decades as a cleansing agent. They produce a deep, rich foam with excellent stability that helps dissolve even the toughest soils and oils on dishes. They are obtained from the roots and leaves of soapwort plants which yields a phytochemical with a skin-softening, anti-irritant effect. The natural product retains water and can be added to food to establish or maintain moisture levels. Saponins can be used in bread, cereal, snacks, soup mixes, pasta products, pet foods, vegetables, and grain-based meals.

Saponins are produced by plants to help protect them against predators. There are different types of saponins. Some saponins have a foaming effect when in contact with water, which is how they work to clean cells. Other types of saponins are absorbed through the skin, to help the body eliminate toxins. They are known to have a large number of biological effects due to their surfactant properties (Kadam & Prabhasankar, 2010).

Saponins are a family of triterpenoid glycosides distributed abundantly in seed plants like legumes, cereal grains, and medicinal herbs that have been widely studied for their effects on human health. Saponins possess diverse pharmacological activities, including antihypertensive, hypolipidemic, antidiabetic, choleretic, and immunosuppressant effects. They belong to a category of plant defenses called triterpenoids. Saponins are widely distributed in herbs, shrubs, and trees. Saponin present groups include many chemical structures that areomers for each other, so people use them as food additives and medicine ingredients.

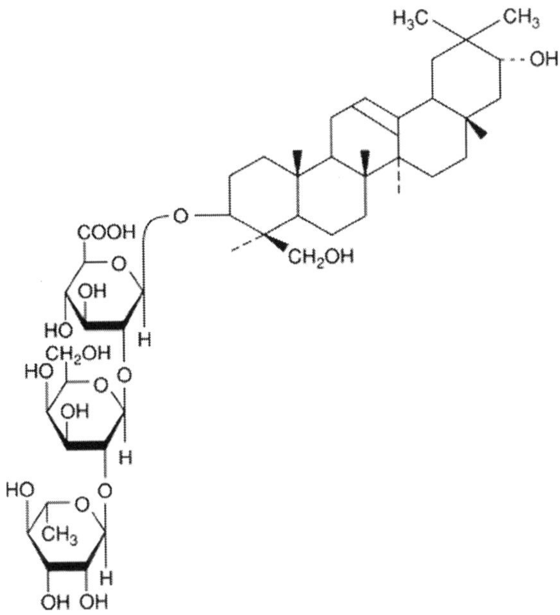

Figure 7.12: The structure of Saponin.

This natural product is extracted from more than 1,400 plant species but is most commonly found in soapwort. Saponins are used by herbalists and practitioners of alternative medicine in the belief that they have medicinal properties. This belief is based primarily on a folkloristic understanding of how saponins are said to act in the body and are not supported by any clinical studies or other forms of evidence-based practice. There is currently insufficient scientific evidence to support health claims made for saponins in alternative medicine. Nor can it be assumed that what is true for one saponin will necessarily be true for all others (Jacob *et al.*, 2020).

The natural products are organic macromolecular glycosides, widely distributed in the plant kingdom and have been used for thousands of years, mainly as food additives to reduce cholesterol. They are also employed at low concentrations (1 mM) as adjuvant immunostimulators to enhance the immune responses when combined with bacterial or viral antigens and in anti-fungal agents.

History of Saponins

Saponins were widely found in medical communities where the benefits of their anti-viral, anti-bacterial, and anti-fungal properties have made them front-line defense in the fight against diseases. Today, modern scientists are studying how saponins can be applied to a wide range of applications beyond traditional medicinal use.

In the early days, they were used for cleansing and liturgical ceremonies. Saponins were accidentally discovered when people tried to turn the roots of the soapwort plant into soap. What they found was that this plant produced a foam that lathered extremely well. It wasn't until later that scientists named this foam, Saponin. The soapberry tree (*Sapindus mukorossi*, syn. *S. Chinensis*) is a tree native to East Asia and introduced to other parts of the world (Ibrahim *et al.*, 2015). It bears fruit that is inedible to humans but contains saponins, especially the glycerides of sapogenin and several related triterpenoid saponins known as sapotoxins.

Occurrence; Saponins are a large and diverse collection of compounds with nature. They are widely distributed in the plant kingdom, particularly in plants such as triterpene and steroid glycosides. Saponin glycoside has been reported to contain steroids including b-sitosterol, stigmasterol, and cholesterol. In addition, a literature survey shows that their greatest concentrations have been reported from higher plants, including Gymnema, Quillaja bark, and Yucca leaves.

Chemistry and biosynthesis behind saponins

Saponins, a group of compounds with varying structural features, exhibit several biological activities. The saponin structure is characterized by a glycosylated aglycone linked by an oxygen bridge to a saccharide and having either one or two hydroxy groups in the sapogenin molecule. Saponins occur naturally in many plant species, with certain species containing as much as 8% of the total dry weight of saponins. Palmaceae, Solanaceae, Fabaceae, and Lamiaceae are the most common families intensively investigated for their saponin content. In addition to plants and seeds, saponins also have been isolated from algae macrofungi, lichens, sponges, and terrestrial invertebrates (Yousuf *et al*., 2021).

Saponins as plant-derived compounds are used in industries as antigenic agents, plant protectants, and surfactants. It has the amphipathic property and is important in terms of its nutritional, pharmaceutical, and commercial properties. Its mode of action plays an important role in many industries such as detergent, food, beverage, cosmetic, pharmaceutical, and plant protection. There are two general classifications of saponin which are aglycone saponins and glycosidically bound saponins known as glycosides. Alcohol is required to obtain saponin, which is done by acid precipitation or solvent extraction. The chemical structure of saponin stimulated research into their isolation, purification, Physico-chemical properties, stability, and biosynthesis. Saponins are synthesized via a complex pathway where a large number of enzymes are involved; they are transported via the phloem to gain certain specific functions (e.g., defense and communication). Saponins have been used with anti-cancer and anti-HIV effects in medicine for years. The toxicity of various extract concentrations must be determined to prevent any negative effects of using saponins in medicine.

Functions and utilization of saponins

Saponins have low toxicity to the human body and are a kind of foam generator with strong stability. It has the effect of lowering surface tension, emulsifying, dispersing, and foaming.

7.1.7 Steroids

Steroids are natural products that contain virtually no calories and are fat-free, low in sodium, and an excellent source of fiber. This product is made from four, naturally occurring steroids that are necessary for life. It works by relieving symptoms such as swelling, pain, and allergic-type reactions. Steroids decrease the body's natural defensive response and reduce symptoms such as swelling and allergic-type reactions.

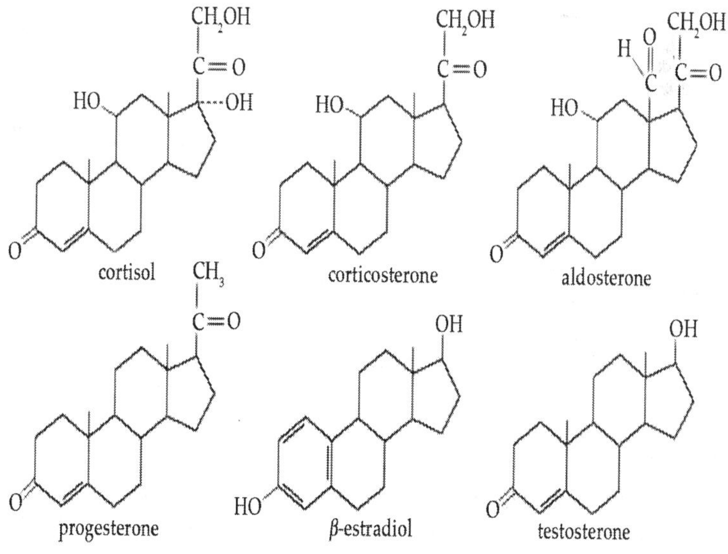

Figure 7.13: The structure of steroids.

It is based on the chemical structure of opiates, especially oxycodone derivatives, which are found in plants such as the peony. Peony is often cultivated as food or ornamental plants in Asia and Europe, while opium is produced mainly in Asia. Steroids have been used for centuries as food preservatives. They are also used as a drug against many diseases, especially cardiovascular disease. The main objective of steroidal products is to reduce inflammation and pain due to excessive use of the muscles (Walker *et al.*, 2015).

We all know that steroids are used by athletes to enhance performance. What you won't hear, however, is that many of these steroid users develop respiratory problems, including the collapse of the lungs. Steroids can also cause stunted growth in younger athletes. Steroids can also cause an absence of menstruation in young women and this is especially dangerous if taken by pregnant women with its potential to cause birth defects such as ovarian cysts. Steroids contain a unique amino acid profile that specifically increases protein synthesis, cellular volumization, and IGF-1 output.

As a drug, it is a perfectly legal drug and it's used as a supplement, just like any other supplement on the market. But it has a very special power when it comes to muscle growth. It is one of the most powerful stimulants of muscle growth that there is. As such, it's extremely effective in building muscle mass but it also has some serious side effects if you take too much of it for too long (Turner & Thompson, 2013). Naturally, steroids are used as a hormone that is derived from Cholesterol. It is also a natural product found in animals, plants, and other living organisms.

History of steroids

The history and diversity of steroids as a natural product are not widely known. It can date back to ancient times, when it was used as a medication for a variety of illnesses, including arthritis and acne. The plant steroid berberine has been found to help treat certain types of diabetes (Vanbergen & Initiative, 2013). It is also known to improve blood flow and circulation. Phytosterols are defined and classified based on the biosynthetic pathway revealed by their distribution in nature. The structural diversity of phytosterols is highlighted, with terpenes and other compounds being transformed into steroidal saponins from which steroids can be extracted and new sterol precursors isolated.

Oral steroids have been used for millennia by many cultures, which can be seen in historical texts. Their uses are still prevalent today in what constitutes a natural plant-derived product. In the 1990s and 2000s, the steroid controversy aroused tremendous public concern. In some parts of the world, professional contests and even physical exercises involving combat sports (MMA, wrestling kolos games) were banned because of their possible use of prohibited substances. Even some countries discussed the prohibition of all other sports events. The World Anti-Doping Agency was formed in 1999 by the International Olympic Committee. In 2000, the U.S. Government began prosecution of Barry Bonds for violation of the Controlled Substances Act because it was "a significant step towards the day when all athletes use a genuine health product."

Chemistry and biosynthesis behind steroids

Interestingly, the shape of the carbon atoms in a steroid molecule has similarities to the cross-section of a bicycle chain. Steroids are a large group of organic compounds that mainly show hydrophobic and gender effects and have similar cyclic structures. Steroids are more different in physicochemical properties, such as polarity and solubility. The intramolecular cyclization of an unsaturated side chain acts to produce a ring structure in natural steroids. All natural steroids are chiral. Chirality can be deduced with the use of a mirror and a basic steroid skeleton.

Anabolic Steroids or anabolic androgenic steroids are synthetic derivatives of testosterone. Both synthetic and natural steroids share androgenic as well as anabolic effects. Anabolism is the process by which organisms construct proteins from amino acids; catabolism is the breakdown of proteins into their constituent amino acids and energy for cellular processes (Tang et al., 2020). Androgens are steroid hormones that stimulate the development and maintenance of male sex characteristics, including growth and maturation of the prostate, seminal vesicles, penis, and scrotum in addition to the development of secondary sexual characteristics such as pubic, facial, and body hair.

Steroidogenesis

Steroidogenesis is the term used for over 200 metabolic reactions that involve a series of chemical reactions converting cholesterol into other steroid hormones, including testosterone and estrogen. Cholesterol is present in every cell of your body and plays a key role in its function. Steroidogenesis occurs in the endoplasmic reticulum within cells of your adrenal glands, gonads (ovaries and testes), brain, adipose tissue, and liver. Because of this specialization in different tissues, cholesterol levels are unique to each individual—they even differ between men and women, as well as change throughout your lifetime. Steroid onset time depends on which steroid it is, and how much sex hormone binding globulin there is that normally binds with your steroids. This means you can't count on going through puberty at a set age due to differences between you and your peers or depending on when you started puberty. However, this makes sense because puberty is hormonally driven which makes nonsense of using predetermined ages to describe it.

Functions of steroids

Today, more and more people are opting to use a natural alternative to traditional prescription drugs. Steroids help to build muscle and increase strength by increasing natural testosterone production. Steroids are present in the human body and are a product of male and female sex hormones. Research states that sterols provide a healthy amount of cholesterol to the body along with other health benefits, such as increased cellular energy (Acosta-Estrada *et al.,* 2021).

Steroids are very famous in the sports field and fitness programs. They improve our physical performance to a great extent and provide us with various kinds of benefits such as muscular strength, good endurance, fast recovery from injuries, etc. Steroids can also aid you in getting the perfect body shape. Overall, steroids make the best combination for increasing physical strength.

Within the human body, however, these substances can attach themselves to different proteins, including one called SHBG (sex hormone binding globulin). When they attach themselves to this specific protein, it stops some testosterone from being active and free in the body. Effects of steroids on fertility seem to work in several ways and as yet are not fully understood. A simple example would be that it might suppress the normal function of luteinizing hormone in the male. However, this would not cause infertility but lower sperm counts and other symptoms. More subtle at the biochemical level is the disruption of intracellular signaling pathways controlling spermatogenesis and this is currently a major focus of study.

7.1.8 Flavonoids

Flavonoids are natural products from plant sources that may support heart health. Flavonoid molecules are the largest polyphenolic group and account for approximately 40% of all plant metabolites. There are more than 4000 kinds of flavonoids, which can be divided into six categories according to their structures: flavones, flavonols, isoflavones, flavanones, anthocyanidins, and retinol. Flavonoid is a secondary metabolite of plants. Scientists are interested in studying these chemicals because they believe that if we can find their effects of them in plant form, we may believe that they possibly do the same thing when consumed by humans (Stintzing & Carle, 2004).

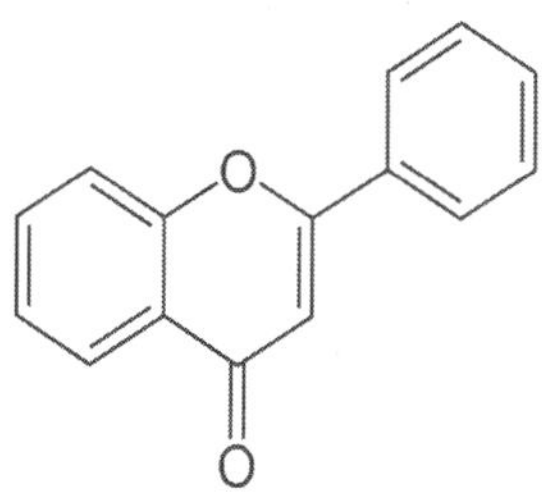

Figure 7.14: The structure of flavonoid.

History and diversity of flavonoids

Flavonoids are widely distributed in the vegetable kingdom. They have long been of interest for their biological activities and culinary applications, but, more recently, flavonoids have also been investigated concerning their ability to use solar energy. Flavonoid biosynthesis has been studied in great detail at the molecular level and many different genes have been identified that contribute to this complex pathway. Recent work has also shed light on the evolution of these compounds and shown that they differ considerably between angiosperms and gymnosperms.

Chemistry and biosynthesis behind flavonoids

Flavonoids have been receiving more and more attention because of their diverse functions, both physiological and pathological. However, the biogenesis and molecular diversity of flavonoids are still poorly understood. These compounds exhibit a variety of biological activities, such as anticancer activity, and anti-inflammatory and antioxidant properties among others. Flavones are characterized by a 5 or 6-member ring containing two methoxy groups, at least one being attached to the 3-carbon in position 3 on the B-ring. This biosynthesis is divided into two major branches that have been studied from different points of view: the phenylpropanoid and the mevalonate pathways (Shipp & Abdel-Aal, 2010).

Flavonoids are the most common subclass of polyphenols in nature. They are usually characterized by a heterocyclic aromatic core, from which two phenolic hydroxyl moieties and a sugar moiety are derived. Flavonoids are a natural product of polyphenol rings which are responsible for the vivid colors in plants. One example is deoxypodophyllotoxin, an alkaloid widely occurring in plants, especially in Podophyllum. Deoxypodophyllotoxin is a precursor of etoposide, a widely used anti-cancer drug. Besides, its alleviating effect on HIV replication has been demonstrated. As it is easily accessible by chemical synthesis but mainly produced by plant cell suspension cultures, its biosynthesis has been subject to intense study. Its 9-O-methyl ether podophyllotoxin is present in the root of the American May Apple (*Podophyllum peltatum*). Macrocarpa A and B represent macrocyclic lignans from *Magnolia grandiflora* that were shown to exhibit potent growth inhibitory activities against various cancer cell lines The structure and biosynthesis of podophyllotoxin, deoxypodophyllotoxin, macrocarpa A and B are compared to illustrate the chemistry and biosynthesis of flavonoids.

Flavonoids are polyphenolic compounds synthesized by plants and are considered to be one of the most important groups of natural pigments. The individual units that make up these polymers have been determined through extensive study, which has facilitated a comprehensive analysis of the structure-function relationship (Sharma *et al.,* 2021). While the coloration and aroma levels depend on various factors (genetic, environmental, etc), other properties such as anti-oxidant, anti-inflammatory, and anti-microbial are inherent to these complex molecules.

Functions of flavonoids

Flavonoids have a wide range of beneficial effects, from the protection of cell membranes to the regulation of the secretion of hormones. Flavonoids act as potent antioxidants and free radical scavengers which help protect against chronic diseases. This formula of potent antioxidants, including flavonoids, plays a major role in boosting immunity, protecting you from free radicals that attack and damage healthy cells and can even help regulate blood sugar levels.

Flavonoids are powerful antioxidants that have anti-inflammatory properties and can help fight oxidative stress. The beneficial effects of drugs that are inactive in their natural form are often due to metabolic activation products (Ambuja & Rajakumar, 2018). In the case of the flavonoid tangeretin, the metabolites methylisoxazolyl-tangeretin and methylisothiazolyl-tangeretin were found in rat plasma, whereas these compounds are absent from the plant. These metabolites proved to be over twice as active as tangeretin as inhibitors of monoamine oxidase (MAO) activity in a cell-free assay.

CHAPTER 8

REASONS PEOPLE ARE TURNING TO NATURAL PRODUCTS

CONTENTS

8.1 INTRODUCTION

The term natural products can be defined in many ways. When most people talk about natural products, they are referring to the products (usual food) that come from the earth, such as milk and honey. However, natural products are any organic compounds found in nature, not man-made when it comes to science (Shipp & Abdel-Aal, 2010). This can include anything from antibiotics and hormones to vitamins and proteins.

In the 1950s, two chemists from the University of Wisconsin, Robert Robinson and Alexander Todd were awarded the Nobel Prize for their work in discovering natural products. This sparked an interest in studying natural products for medicinal uses.

Natural Products were first discovered by ancient cultures who used them for beauty treatments and health remedies. The Egyptians were known for using animal fats, minerals, herbs, and leaves as part of their daily health routines. As centuries passed, different cultures around the world began studying the effects of various natural products on their bodies and environments (Sharma et al., 2021). However, some researchers believe that natural products should only come from plants because they don't have a central nervous system that could affect their behavior, and they don't have a soul that could make them feel pain when they are harvested for their chemicals.

Natural products are used in the food industry as sweeteners, flavorings, fragrances, and preservatives. They are also used as medicines to treat human diseases. The idea behind using natural substances isn't a new one: civilizations have been using plant-based materials for thousands of years. But since the Industrial Revolution in 18th century Britain, we've seen an increase in large companies creating products with fewer and fewer natural ingredients. With this change, there's been a rise in concerns about the quality and safety of these products. Companies started to notice this concern and began marketing their products as "natural" again. The only problem: there weren't any laws or regulations to back up these claims. Nowadays, companies are required to provide evidence supporting their claims of all-natural products.

Natural products are a broad category of chemicals that are produced by living organisms like plants. They can be divided into four classes: terpenes and terpenoids, alkaloids, phenolic compounds, Steroids, Polyketides, and fatty acid derivatives (Rochfort, 2005). The first group of common natural products is alkaloids. Alkaloids are found in more than twenty percent of all plants. They can be classified by their chemical structure as either purines or pyridines. One great example of an alkaloid is caffeine, which is a purine that stimulates cell activity and speeds up the central nervous system.

Another common type of natural product is a terpene. Terpenes are organic compounds that contain organic hydrocarbons and make up an important part of human life. About forty percent of all known organic compounds are terpenes or derivatives thereof. Terpenes are very important in the pharmaceutical industry because they have antibacterial properties and can help with brain and muscle function. Terpenoids are compounds that are derived from terpenes, which are hydrocarbons. These compounds are made up of isoprene units and can be classified by their number of isoprene units. For example, sesquiterpenes have 15 carbons and three isoprene units, and diterpenes have 20 carbons and four isoprene units (Ribeiro *et al.*, 2019). There are two major types of terpenoids: hemiterpenoids which are one isoprene unit, which is not common in biology, and linear terpenoids with two or more isoprene units. Phenolics are compounds that contain 2 benzene rings with a ketone group attached to one of them; they were first discovered while studying the negative effects of coal tars on people's skin.

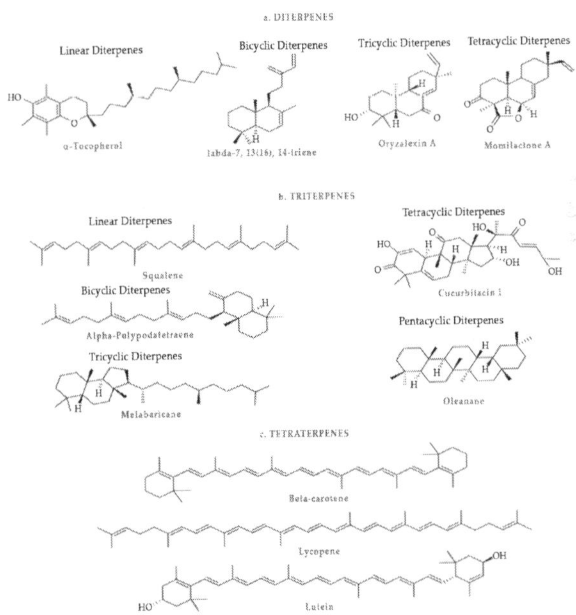

Figure 8.1: An image showing the chemical structure of terpenes which is a natural product.

(Source: Ninkuu V, Zhang L, et, al., 2021)

Steroids are best known for their use in sports, where they can improve strength and endurance, but they can also be used to treat several conditions like arthritis and asthma, and they're even quite beneficial to your skin's health.

Polyketides derive from fatty acid precursors, which consist of acetyl-CoA subunits. They tend to include aromatic rings in their structure, which makes them a major class of secondary metabolites. Polyketides can be cyclic or acyclic, with the cyclic polyketides derived either from iterative polyketide synthases or type I polyketide synthases. The acyclic forms are made by non-ribosomal peptide synthases with mixed biosynthetic pathways.

Natural products are everywhere these days. It's no longer enough to know they're sustainable and environmentally friendly. Sourced from natural ingredients in that the product is made from ingredients that can all be found in nature without further processing. Eco-friendly packaging in that the product's packaging is recyclable or biodegradable, thus not adding to the world's landfill problems. Safe and non-toxic whereby there are no harsh chemicals in the product that could cause harm to humans or animals when ingested or inhaled (Proksch *et al.*, 2003). Ethically sourced whereby all of the ingredients for the product have been obtained and/or produced without harming people or animals. Cruelty-free in the sense that no animals were harmed in the process of creating the product and/or any of its ingredients.

Natural beauty whereby the product was created with a focus on making people feel beautiful, comfortable, and confident in their bodies. Organic which are products that have been certified organic are grown without the use of synthetic pesticides, herbicides, or fertilizers. They can't contain genetically modified seeds or organisms (GMOs). The USDA oversees organic certification. Non-GMOs are products that do not include genetically modified organisms (GMOs) or ingredients derived from GMOs. The Non-GMO Project is the largest verifier of product claims for GMO avoidance in the United States and Canada. A vegan product doesn't contain any animal materials or byproducts like meat, eggs, dairy, honey, leather, fur, wool, feathers, silk, beeswax, wool wax, gelatin, carmine, a red pigment from crushed insects, and shellac, a resin secreted by beetles. Veganism is a lifestyle choice that encompasses foods as well as other products like clothing and cosmetics. The Vegan Society trademark is one official way to know a product.

8.2 REASONS FOR TURNING TO NATURAL PRODUCTS

Many people turn to natural products due to allergies or sensitivities created by many of the chemicals in use today. Others are hoping to avoid exposing their families and pets to harsh ingredients. Some believe that natural products can help them reduce their carbon footprint, while others hope for a more environmentally friendly approach to product creation (Pop *et al.*, 2019). Still, others are interested in the potential health benefits of using products with natural ingredients. Finally, some people turn to natural products simply because they feel better about using them since they know that the ingredients will not harm themselves or the environment.

8.3 FUNCTIONS OF NATURAL PRODUCTS

Natural products are an important part of our world. One of the most important functions of natural products is to help keep people healthy. Natural products can be used to treat illnesses, but they can also be used to prevent them altogether. Another function of natural products is that they can be used for food. Different countries use different kinds of foods for different reasons. Some do it for taste, some do it for nutrition, and others do it for both. People also use natural products to make their houses look nicer. People like having flowers in their yards and having grass that's always green. This can make a home look better and more appealing. Natural products have many functions; they can be used as a moisturizer, skin tone, or even as a treatment for different skin conditions like eczema and psoriasis. It is also important to note that natural products are cost-effective when it comes to purchasing them. Many natural products have a low toxic potential, which makes them safe to use. They also tend to be biodegradable and non-irritating to the skin and eyes.

In the 1990s, scientists first discovered that primary metabolites, the chemicals responsible for basic functions in an organism, can be used as natural products. Primary metabolites are usually produced in large quantities by an organism. They include amino acids, lipids, and other molecules like sugar, nucleic acids, and vitamins. Another example of a primary metabolite is glutathione peroxidase, a protein enzyme that helps to prevent oxidative damage to cells. Glutathione peroxidase has antioxidant properties and can protect cells from free radicals or other toxins that may cause damage (Odhaib *et al.*, 2021). Some primary metabolites are used in the creation of secondary metabolites, which tend to be more chemically complex than primary metabolites. Since then, their importance has been made more apparent, and several studies have shown that they are integral to plant survival. Primary metabolites have been shown to have a wide range of functions: fragrance molecules, pheromones, and even poisons. Their role as plant hormones is also well-studied. Because they are so important, primary metabolites are produced in large quantities by plants. This makes them easy to obtain and use in our efforts to produce healthy food for the world's population. It's one reason why scientists are so eager to discover new natural products; once we know what a plant naturally produces, we can begin to imitate it in our laboratories. Secondary metabolites are natural products that might have a function in the organism that produces them, but they are not needed to stay alive. While there are many types of secondary metabolites, they all have one thing in common: they are produced by a living organism (Murdoch *et al.,* 2000). Secondary metabolites can be fungicides, antibiotics, or toxins. They can be used as protection against predators, or to help an organism get access to nutrients. Secondary metabolites are often produced by bacteria and fungi, but plants also produce them.

8.4 IMPORTANCE OF BIOSYNTHESIS OF NATURAL PRODUCTS TO PEOPLE

The term, biosynthesis, denotes the process of natural production of a product by living organisms. The biosynthetic processes are highly specific to each organism and require the presence of vital enzymes. The role of biosynthesis in the survival of organisms is enormous as it allows them to produce compounds that they need for their survival to get adapted to their environment (Multari *et al.,* 2015). Biosynthesis is also important for their growth, reproduction, and development.

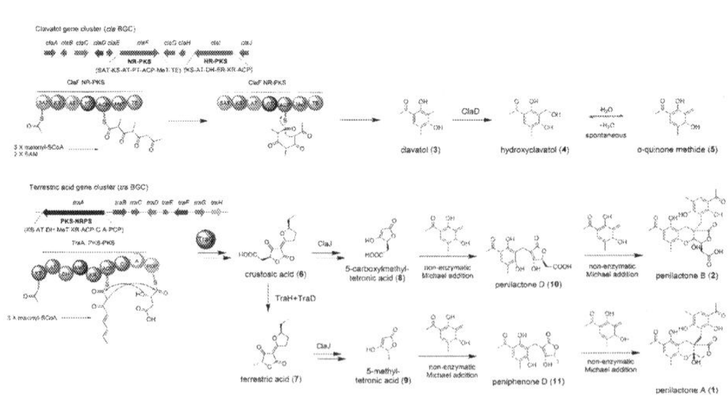

Figure 8.2: An image showing the biosynthesis process of natural products.

(Source: Dai G, Shen Q, et, al., 2022)

Natural products are those produced by nature. They are often produced by plants and animals but they can also be made by various micro-organisms. These products include proteins, vitamins, hormones, and various other organic compounds that are essential for life. Natural products are used widely by humans in different fields such as biotechnology, medicine, agriculture, and food production. Humans utilize natural products in different ways: as medicines or drugs, as dietary supplements, in agricultural applications, in the cosmetics industry, and the food industry. Natural products may be extracted from plants or animals directly or they may be obtained from micro-organisms using various techniques such as fermentation.

8.5 BIOSYNTHESIS OF CARBOHYDRATES

The biosynthesis of carbohydrates as natural products is important to people because they are used in a wide variety of applications. The biosynthesis of carbohydrates is useful in the production of biofuels, food and feed additives, and animal feed. In addition, these processes can be used for making industrial products such as plastics, paper, and textiles (Linares et al., 2017). The production of natural products by these processes can also be used for producing pharmaceuticals and other medical products.

Carbohydrates are produced from plants through processes that include photosynthesis, fermentation, and pyrolysis. These processes use energy from the sun or organic matter such as wood or coal. To get this energy, plants must have access to light, water, and nutrients. When plants are grown under conditions where they do not receive enough light or water, they will not produce enough carbohydrates for their needs.

In addition to using energy from the sun or organic matter, the production process must also use a source of carbon dioxide (CO2). This is necessary because CO2 is a greenhouse gas that contributes to global warming if it is not captured before being emitted into the atmosphere. It can be captured in several ways including burning fossil fuels like coal or oil; burning biomass such as wood chips; capturing CO2 from industries.

The biosynthesis of carbohydrates is crucial to the survival of humans and other organisms. Carbohydrates contain energy that is necessary to fuel cells and carry out various metabolic functions. The most common type of carbohydrate is glucose, which is produced by photosynthesis in plants. In humans, glucose is absorbed into the bloodstream after carbohydrates are consumed (López *et al.*, 2019). In the bloodstream, glucose is used as a source of cellular energy by all human cells, including muscle cells and brain cells. Glucose can also be stored in the liver and then released back into the bloodstream when the body needs more energy.

Biosynthesis occurs when two molecules react to form a new molecule. In this process, one molecule is used as a substrate for another molecule to create a new product. The enzyme amylase breaks down complex carbohydrates into simpler sugars that can then be digested by the body's digestive system. People who suffer from diabetes have trouble regulating their blood sugar levels because they lack sufficient amounts of insulin or cannot use it efficiently enough on their own. It's important to understand how our body processes food so that we can better control our blood sugar levels and avoid health issues such as obesity, cardiovascular disease, cancer, and type II diabetes.

8.6 BIOSYNTHESIS OF FATTY ACIDS AND POLYKETIDES

Polyketides and fatty acids are two important types of natural products which are synthesized by microorganisms and plants. Polyketides can be described as metabolites with a molecular weight greater than 1500 Daltons that contain two or more Ketide units. Polyketides are used for treating a wide range of health problems from bacterial infections to cancer. Fatty acids, also known as lipids, are organic molecules composed of carbon, hydrogen, and oxygen atoms (Karioti et al., 2015). They consist of chains of atoms that contain at least one carboxyl group (-COOH). Many fatty acids are essential nutrients for human survival. This is why the Biosynthesis of fatty acids and polyketides as Natural Products is important to people.

8.7 MEDICAL USES OF NATURAL PRODUCTS

While the advent of modern medicine has brought us many new and exciting medical treatments, some of the most effective medical treatments have been around for centuries. For example, essential oils from plants, known as botanicals, have long been used to treat a wide variety of ailments. Some examples of natural products are berries, grass, animals, rocks, and diamonds. Natural products can be changed in many ways to make useful things for people. Many medicines we use come from plants or animals. People can get medicines from natural products because they understand how the medicines work and what they do to help our bodies.

A number of these natural products work by binding to specific protein targets in the body, which causes a cascade of reactions that can have beneficial effects. These include shikonin and eugenol, which bind to certain tumor cells and cause cell death; capsaicin and curcumin, which are both anti-inflammatory and help fight cancer; and even caffeine from coffee beans, which can stimulate the brain to promote wakefulness (Khorram & Ramezanian, 2021). These natural products also have fewer side effects than traditional prescription drugs. For example, capsaicin is very effective at relieving pain with fewer side effects than prescription painkillers like acetaminophen or opioids.

8.8 THE USE OF NATURAL PRODUCTS AS A SOURCE OF TRADITIONAL MEDICINE

One of the biggest trends in health and wellness for the past few years has been the return to natural, plant-based products for healing. It's not a new concept, many cultures have used plants as a source of traditional medicine for centuries (Karthika & Sureshkumar, 2021). But in recent years, more and more people have turned to herbal remedies as an alternative to over-the-counter or prescription drugs, especially when it comes to treating common ailments like headaches, colds, and menstrual cramps.

And now, these plant-based products are becoming more widely available than ever before. You can find them in your local grocery store or pharmacy alongside other supplements and pain relievers, or even online with just a few clicks. For many people who use them regularly or experimentally, they provide relief without the side effects of pharmaceuticals; and they're often less expensive than traditional medicine too. Natural products are not necessarily better than synthetic alternatives because they can be more complex in composition and can also be subject to variability by factors such as species, cultivation practices, genetic drift, or environmental conditions.

There are many benefits to using natural products over synthetic drugs. One of them is the fact that they were designed by nature through natural selection and genetic mutation over millions of years. This makes them more likely to be effective than synthetic drugs, which can have harmful side effects often since they are not naturally derived or haven't been tested on humans for long enough periods (Jacob *et al.*, 2020). Natural products also tend to be less expensive than man-made medications, since nature doesn't charge for its work.

8.9 THE USE OF NATURAL PRODUCTS AS A SOURCE OF MODERN NATURAL PRODUCT-DERIVED DRUGS

Natural products have been used for thousands of years in the prevention and treatment of diseases. Almost all drugs have been obtained from natural products or are inspired by them. In fact, many of the most important drugs developed to date have come from natural sources. The use of natural products in modern cancer therapy is also increasing, with several natural product-derived drugs currently being used by physicians worldwide.

The use of natural products as a source of modern natural product-derived drugs has increased significantly in recent years. With the advent of technology and industrialization, it has become possible to synthesize many drugs in laboratories that mimic natural products. But natural products are still very important in drug development because they often possess properties that are difficult to synthesize in a lab and easier to create in a biological system (Bulaj *et al.*, 2016). The reason for this increase is mainly due to their high therapeutic potential, which is associated with their high molecular diversity and ability to specifically target molecular targets involved in disease processes. Natural products may be defined as compounds produced by living organisms that have biological activity.

8.10 THE USE OF NATURAL PRODUCTS AS A SOURCE OF LIMITING AND ENABLING FACTORS

The use of natural products as a source of limiting and enabling factors is one of the best ways to ensure that you are getting the most out of your money. There are many benefits to using natural products, but they also have their downsides as well. For many people who do not have the resources or skills to produce their natural products, several companies will provide this service for them. This can be a great way to get started on your project, but you need to make sure that you choose a company that has experience in this field. You should also make sure that you are dealing with someone from the same city or state as yourself.

It's important to remember that these companies will often charge more than if you were to buy the products on your own. Many times, it is possible for you to find natural products at other places as well, but it can sometimes be difficult to get everything that you need in one place. It's always better to buy from someone who knows what they're doing and understands the process better than anyone else does (Ibrahim *et al.*, 2015). In addition, some of these companies will only offer the following: pure natural products in bulk, and they may not even offer any type of guarantee or support after they've been purchased. The natural products that have been used in the past as sources of limiting and enabling factors include the Use of liming agents. Liming agents are compounds that are produced naturally in soils by organisms that inhabit them. They can be produced by plants, fungi, bacteria, or other organisms. Use of organic acids: Organic acids are produced by the action of microorganisms on organic matter such as plants and animals during decomposition. Some organic acids are produced naturally while others are man-made. These include citric acid (found in citrus fruits), malic acid (found in apples), tartaric acid (found in grapes), lactic acid (found in milk), acetic acid (found in vinegar), and oxalic acid (found in spinach). This also includes the use of different kinds of nitrogenous compounds such as ammonia, nitric oxide (NO), or nitrous oxide (N2O).

As limiting factors, natural products are often hard to obtain because of their location or price. There are also several legal restrictions on obtaining these substances, such as the illegal drug trade. In addition, some natural products cannot be synthesized by humans so they must be obtained from nature to be used as medicine. As enabling factors, natural products can be very effective when it comes to treating certain illnesses without causing side effects like other medications might cause (Hou & Xu, 2022). They also tend to cost less than synthetic drugs making them an affordable option for those who cannot afford other types of treatment.

Natural products are a popular source of nutrition in our modern world: many people believe that these products are safer and healthier than products that are created in a laboratory. However, it is important to be aware that not all natural products are safe to use or consume. Some of them may even be dangerous. This is because there are many different types of chemicals contained within natural materials and these chemical reactions can cause serious problems if they occur in an uncontrolled way. To avoid this danger, we need to understand what types of chemicals exist naturally in nature before we start using them. We also need to know the effects that these chemicals may have on us as humans. If we do not take care when choosing our food sources then there is no way for us to prevent any harmful effects from occurring (Hathwar *et al.*, 2012). The first step towards learning about these types of chemical reactions is by researching them on the internet or by reading books about this subject matter at your local library.

8.11 IMPORTANCE OF ISOLATION AND PURIFICATION OF NATURAL PRODUCTS TO GENERAL HUMAN HEALTH

Humans have used natural products for medicinal purposes since the beginning of time. Naturally occurring products from plants and fungi, for example, were used to treat a wide range of diseases. About a third of the drugs we use today were derived from natural products. For example, aspirin was originally derived from willow bark.

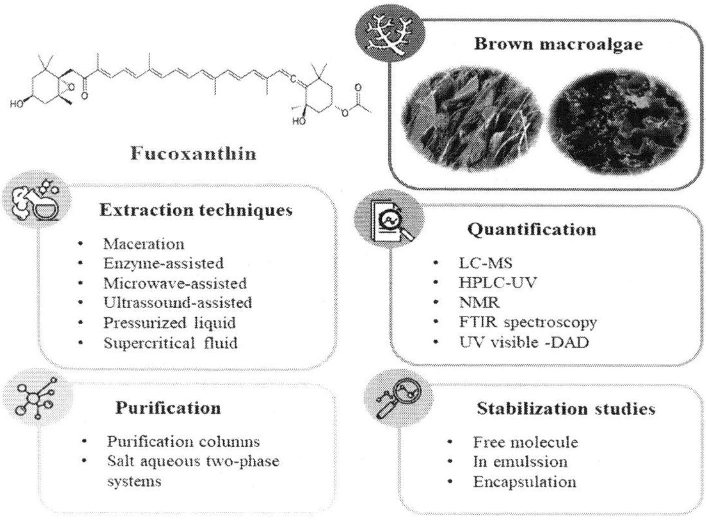

Figure 8.3: An image showing the process of isolation and purification of natural products.

(Source: Lourenço-Lopes C, et, al.,2020)

Isolation and purification of natural products have been practiced since ancient times. As with so many other technologies, it began in the Middle East during the Bronze Age. Ancient Mesopotamian alchemists were working with a few dozen compounds, mostly involving sulfur and salt. Salt was one of the most important substances of ancient times: without it, food quickly spoils, and they didn't have any way to preserve it. Sulfur was also an important substance for them to work with: they used it in wine production and for mummification practices. So it's no surprise that these two substances would be the first to come under scrutiny (Ferreira & Nunes, 2019).

After these early experiments in the Middle East, isolating and purifying natural products would become a central part of Greek and Roman science for centuries to come. For example, in the 3rd century BC, Theophrastus wrote about his observations on how different plants grow from soil that contains different amounts of salt a classic experiment in plant physiology. In the 1st century AD, Pliny the Elder wrote Naturalis Historia, which is still a foundational text in many sciences today, and parts of that book are dedicated to describing various substances used by chemists at the time. But scientists are still discovering new techniques to isolate and purify natural products. In the past, plants were used as a source of medicine. They usually had fruit, roots, or leaves that could be used for medicinal purposes. However, it was difficult to find the right plant because there were so many different types of plants. Scientists discovered that some plants had more than one beneficial component. They also learned that some components were toxic or harmful to humans. They then started looking for ways to separate the harmful components from the beneficial ones. They also found out that they could use heat to separate these components. The process was called distillation and it allowed them to separate oils from water and alcohol from water.

Historically, people didn't know what specific chemicals in these natural products were responsible for their medicinal effects. However, scientists have learned that they could isolate and purify these chemicals to make them more potent and effective medicines. For example, aspirin is a chemical isolated from willow bark that has medicinal properties. Recently scientists have been able to synthesize aspirin in the lab instead of isolating it from natural sources.

Natural products are everywhere in our everyday lives. They're in the food we eat, the medicine we take, and the plants we use to decorate our homes. From ibuprofen to essential oils, they play a vital role in our health and well-being (Francesconi, 2007). Before they can make it into your medicine cabinet or cupboard, they go through a painstaking series of steps to get them there.

Isolation and purification are necessary to ensure the safety and effectiveness of any natural product that is meant for human consumption or use. To start, scientists must first find a way to obtain the desired substance from its source. Then, they must extract it using different chemicals or solvents depending on what type of material is being used as a source; plant, fungus, animal, among others. Next, they must extract the desired substance from the extraction mixture by isolating it from any other substances that may have been extracted. Once these steps have been done correctly, scientists will be able to purify the product for human use. This is important because if you don't isolate and purify your product correctly then it could be dangerous or ineffective for human use.

8.12 THE BENEFITS OF SEMISYNTHESIS OF NATURAL PRODUCTS

While synthetic processes have been the go-to method for producing natural products, semisynthesis has emerged as a popular alternative in recent years. Semisynthesis relies on the use of natural products as starting materials to achieve the desired end product. The process is highly advantageous because it allows scientists to produce complicated compounds that would be difficult or impossible to create using synthesized materials alone. In addition to its ability to make the production of complicated compounds possible, the semisynthesis process also offers several other benefits (Fabani *et al.*, 2013). These benefits include: Cost savings. Using semisynthesis significantly reduces production costs for natural products because it often requires fewer steps than synthesis and does not require advanced equipment. Because of this, businesses can expect to see a significant improvement in their bottom line when they choose semisynthesis over synthesis for natural product production.

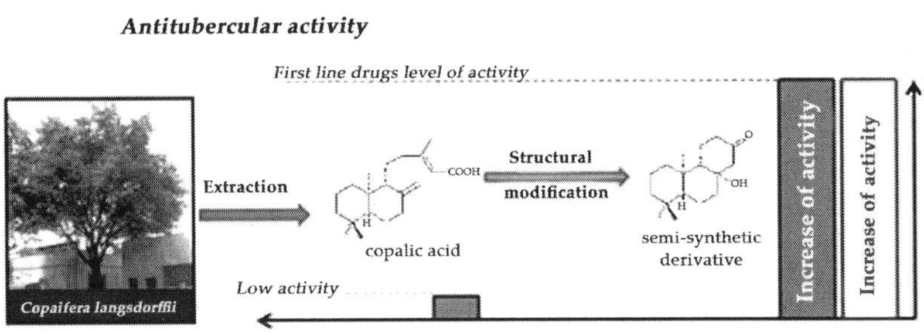

Figure 8.4: An illustration of the semisynthesis of natural products.

(Source: Matos PM, Mahoney B, et, al., 2015)

Because it involves fewer steps, the semisynthesis process is often much more efficient than the synthesized approach to making natural products, especially in cases where new drugs are being developed. This increased efficiency can help businesses produce more items per day, which will ultimately lead to greater profits and stronger customer satisfaction. Semisynthesis is generally less harmful to the environment because it uses fewer chemicals than other methods of production (Dixon & Sumner, 2003). It can be accomplished with less equipment and less time because it does not require extensive processing or refinement. Third, semisynthesis is an innovative way to produce chemical products that are naturally occurring in nature. The result is a product with many benefits for consumers and businesses alike.

8.13 THE BENEFITS OF TOTAL SYNTHESIS OF NATURAL PRODUCTS

Natural products are a key source of new medicines and chemical tools for use in research. While isolated natural products are valuable, total synthesis can provide a more reliable and practical means of obtaining these compounds. Synthesis allows the production of pure material, which is important when working with complex structures that may be challenging to isolate from a single species, i.e., those with multiple stereocenters. The synthesis also allows for the production of analogs that can be used to study structure-function relationships, as well as the production of scarce natural products that have been identified but are not available in sufficient quantities.

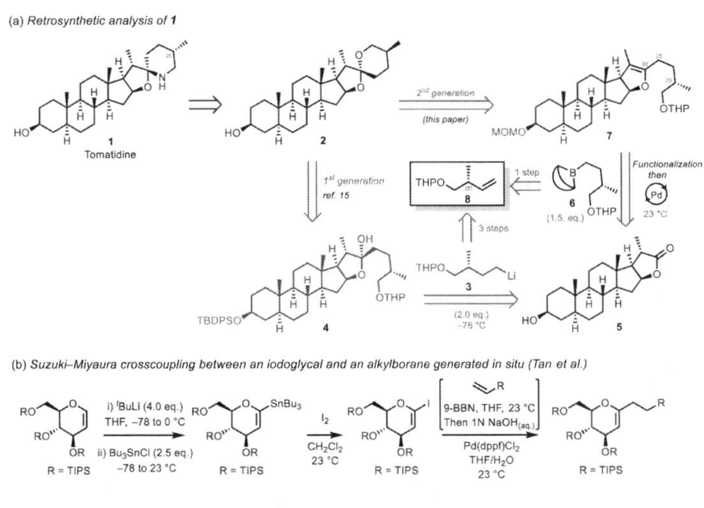

Figure 8.5: An illustration of the total synthesis of natural products.

(Source: Normandin C, and Boudreault P-L. 2021)

Synthesis of natural products dates back to the mid-1800s when William Henry Perkin invented the first synthetic dye. This paved the way for other scientists to experiment with synthesizing natural products, an area of chemistry that had previously been dominated by extraction from organic materials like plants and animals. After World War II, synthetic chemistry became much more widespread and began to center around practical applications like drug development. In the 1950s and 1960s, research began to suggest that some synthetic chemicals were dangerous or even carcinogenic (Da Silva et al., 2016). The public began to demand more "natural" products in response. As a result, companies began to explore new ways of creating beauty products without relying on harmful synthetics like phthalates or parabens. Since then, chemists have been able to invent new synthetic drugs at a much faster rate than they could with natural products alone.

Natural products often have very complex stereochemistry, which can be difficult to analyze and study through isolation alone. Total synthesis allows chemists to explore all possible stereoisomers of a molecule. This can reveal information about how minute differences in structure impact biological activity or other properties of the molecule.

Total synthesis can also offer a more economical and reliable means of obtaining molecules for research or drug development. In some cases, the source of a natural product may be difficult to cultivate or obtain in large quantities. Additionally, isolating compounds from their native sources requires extraction and purification steps that can be expensive and time-consuming.

The benefits of the total synthesis of natural products are numerous. The first is that we can produce as many of the products as we want. If a certain product is in high demand, we can make more. If a certain product is not in high demand, we can make less of it. Total synthetic production of these products allows us to easily adjust our production volume to match consumer demand. In addition, total synthetic production gives us much more control over the process (Dayan *et al.*, 2009). We can make changes to the production process at any time, and if a change causes too many problems or does not work out, we can easily reverse it and try again. This allows us to experiment with different methods of producing natural products, which allows for greater innovation and creativity in this field. Finally, total synthetic production reduces waste. When a company uses traditional methods to produce natural products, it may end up throwing out some materials that are not used in the final product. Synthetic production allows us to use all of the materials we have on hand to create natural products without having any leftovers or scraps go unused.

8.14 THE BENEFITS OF SYMMETRY OF NATURAL PRODUCTS AS A FORM OF SYNTHESIS

The symmetry of natural products as a form of synthesis is a method of performing chemical reactions on organic compounds, in which the substrate is mixed with an acid or base and heated, forming a salt. The salt reacts with the substrate to give an ester or amide. This process can be repeated until the desired product is obtained. The main benefit of this type of synthesis is that it allows products to be made in a way that is very cost-effective and efficient.

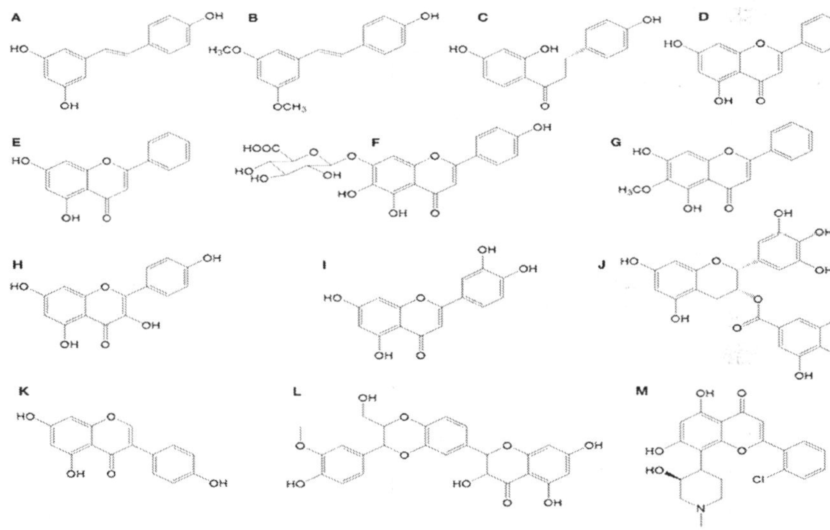

Figure 8.6: An illustration of the symmetry of natural products.

(A) Resveratrol, (B) pterostilbene, (C) isoliquiritigenin, (D) apigenin, (E) chrysin, (F) quercetin, (G) oroxylin, (H) kaempferol, (I) genistein, (J) flavopiridol, (K) silibinin, (L) scutellarin, (M) EGCG.

(Source: Redondo-Blanco S, Fernández J., et al., 2017)

The synthesis of natural products is the process of combining two or more compounds to form a new compound. Many types of synthesis exist. These include one-dimensional, two-dimensional, and three-dimensional syntheses. The most common type of synthesis is one-dimensional synthesis. One-dimensional synthesis is similar to the chemical reaction between two molecules. In this process, an electron from one molecule transfers to another molecule to form a new one. However, there are some differences between this kind of synthesis and the other types. For example, in one-dimensional synthesis, only one reaction takes place at a time. This means that there are no side reactions such as oxidation or reduction reactions occurring during the process (Caporgno & Mathys, 2018).

The second type of synthetic method is called two-dimensional synthesis. In this type of synthetic method, two molecules can react together to form a new compound that has different properties than either molecule separately. For example, if you mix hydrogen peroxide and water in equal amounts then they will react together to make a hydrogen peroxide solution that contains both molecules dissolved in it.

8.15 NATURAL PRODUCTS AS ECOFRIENDLY TO PEOPLE

Natural products are the safest and most eco-friendly products for human beings. Nowadays, natural products are in high demand as there is an awareness among people to protect the environment. Natural products have many benefits such as they have fewer side effects when compared to chemical products. Natural products can be also used for skin care as well as hair care. Moreover, natural products are environmentally friendly, as they will not cause any pollution to the environment.

Natural products have been proven to be a better alternative to chemicals in terms of safety. They are also better for the environment because they're made from renewable sources like plants and animals that grow naturally without being affected by human interference, which means they don't need as many resources or energy inputs compared with petroleum-based synthetic materials (Cassani *et al.,* 2020). These types of products also tend to last longer than their synthetic counterparts due to their high-quality ingredients and lack of preservatives and additives which can break down over time making them less effective at doing what you need them for.

People are conscious of environmental protection and that is why they prefer more of natural products more than chemical products. Natural products are free from chemicals and fillers, so it is safer to use on the skin. Natural products can also be used for weight loss, as they contain more herbs that help in fat burning. Another benefit of using natural products is that they do not cause any side effects when compared with chemical products, so you can use these natural products without worrying about side effects.

8.16 RELEVANCE OF STRUCTURAL THEORIES OF NATURAL PRODUCTS TO PEOPLE

Natural products include organic compounds, inorganic compounds, and life forms. Organic chemistry assigns the classification of natural products to organic compounds. Inorganic compounds are often described as natural products, but they may or may not be categorized as such by chemists. In addition, living organisms are also classified as natural products. Living organisms contain many chemical substances that are vital for survival and that can be found in nature.

The structural theories of natural products were developed to help scientists understand how these types of structures relate to each other. These theories have been used in many different fields including medicine, biotechnology, and environmental science. They have also been used to determine the best way to classify natural products based on their structures (Yousuf & Siddiqui, 2021). The structural theories of natural products have a lot to offer us. They are a useful way of understanding the world around us, and they can help us to understand our place in it.

8.17 RELEVANCE OF ORGANIC AND NATURAL PRODUCTS CHEMISTRY TO PEOPLE

The advances in Organic and Natural Products Chemistry have been immense over the past century, but many people are unaware of how their lives have been positively impacted. Here is a brief overview of some of the ways this branch of chemistry has influenced our daily lives: Pharmaceuticals: The drugs we take to treat illness or alleviate pain often contain organic compounds that have been synthesized in the lab. These chemicals are researched and tested before they are used in products we use every day. Cosmetics: The cosmetics industry relies heavily on chemical synthesis to provide us with products that keep our hair healthy, our skin glowing, and our teeth clean. Clothes: Natural fibers like cotton or wool require processing before they can be used to make clothes, and the processing plants often rely on organic compounds to clean and dye the fibers so they can be soft against our skin. Foods: The foods we eat rely on organic compounds for preservation, coloring, flavoring, and many other purposes (Walker *et al.*, 2015).

8.18 NATURAL PRODUCTS AS CHEMICAL-FREE

Many people are so used to buying products that are created in labs and contain chemicals that they are unaware of how many amazing products are made from natural ingredients. When you choose natural products, you get to experience them in their purest form, without any negative side effects. When you buy natural products, you're getting exactly what's promised on the label. Natural products don't have added preservatives or artificial ingredients that can produce harmful side effects. If a product claims to be made with lavender, for example, then it is made with lavender, nothing more. You can trust that the product does exactly what it says it does.

Many of the chemicals and other substances found in other beauty products can irritate your skin and cause problems if used over time. It's important to know that all-natural beauty products will not leave behind any residue or damage your skin because they lack harmful additives (Vanbergen & Initiative, 2013). This makes them ideal for people with sensitive skin who need to avoid harsh chemicals and synthetic colors or fragrances. Because natural beauty products don't contain harmful chemicals, they won't be doing any damage.

8.19 BENEFITS OF NATURAL PRODUCTS AS HANDMADE TO PEOPLE

Handmade products have a certain touch that makes them stand out among the rest of the beauty products on the market. Natural ingredients are one of the most important reasons why you should start using handmade products for your skin and hair care needs. While there are tons of synthetic ingredients available on the market, natural ingredients can be found in nature. This means that you do not need to spend a lot of money on expensive synthetic products.

Natural ingredients are also much safer to use on your skin and hair than synthetic ingredients since they do not contain any harmful chemicals or toxins. The fact that these natural ingredients are found in nature makes it much easier for them to be absorbed into your skin and hair, making them more effective at providing nourishment to your skin and hair. Natural ingredients such as tea tree oil and Aloe Vera gel have been used by many cultures throughout history to treat all kinds of ailments, including acne and other skin conditions (Turner & Thompson, 2013). Organic products have also been known to help people with allergies because they do not contain any harsh chemicals or fragrances.

Using handmade soap, shampoo, and skincare products is a great way to support your immune system. It's all about the antioxidants and vitamins in our natural ingredients. When it comes to natural skincare, there are many benefits to using handmade products instead of mass-produced ones. Some of the best reasons to use natural bath and body products include: They can help reduce wrinkles and fine lines naturally. They may help reduce redness, blotchiness, and inflammation of the skin. They may help heal scars, burns, stretch marks, and other skin problems. They may help fight acne by killing bacteria on the surface of the skin without over-drying it out. They help moisturize dry skin without clogging pores and causing breakouts as petroleum-based lotions do! With our lotions, your skin will feel silky smooth all day.

Since handmade items take a lot of time and effort to produce, they are usually more expensive than mass-produced items. If you're looking for something that will last longer than most other things, then handmade is something worth considering.

8.20 BENEFITS OF NATURAL PRODUCTS AS SUSTAINABLE PRODUCTS

Sustainable products are important for many reasons, but one of the most important is being able to sustain healthy ecosystems. Ecosystems that have been disrupted by unsustainable activity have a hard time supporting the plants and animals that live there, which can lead to the extinction of some species and even local losses of biodiversity. Sustainability is also important because it's something we can do now, we don't have to wait until some unknown point in the future when we might be able to undo the damage caused by our unsustainable practices.

Natural products in particular are great because they're made from natural materials that haven't been processed using chemical or energy-intensive processes. This means they're less likely to contribute to pollution and habitat loss. Natural products are biodegradable, renewable, recyclable, and non-toxic. They are also often grown without pesticides or other chemicals (Tang *et al.,* 2020). Biodegradable natural products decompose naturally and safely into the soil without leaving toxic residue. Renewable resources are those that are replenished on a human time scale, such as bamboo and hemp. Recycled materials take less energy to process than new materials and reduce our dependence on raw materials. Non-toxic natural products don't contain synthetic chemicals or additives, which pose health risks.

8.21 BENEFITS OF NATURAL PRODUCTS AS NON-FACTORY MADE PRODUCTS

Natural products are awesome. They're all-natural and made by hand in small batches, not in a factory like those other products, which we're not going to name here but you know who they are. They smell better, too because they have no chemicals in them. You can tell because they don't smell like chemicals! That's how you can tell real natural products from fake natural products, but you should still check the label to be sure.

We all want to live greener lives and take care of our planet and natural products help us do that. When you buy natural products, you're helping the earth by supporting local small businesses that care about their community and environment. If you buy other kinds of products, then you're just supporting big business, you know, the kinds whose names are on buildings downtown (Stintzing & Carle, 2004). But if you buy natural products, then your money is going back into your community which helps everyone. Natural products are also better for you than those factory-made things, which means they will make your hair and skin feel better than ever before.

Conclusion

Natural products are a great way to keep your body and soul healthy and happy. Finding natural solutions to everyday problems is a healthy, sustainable way to care for yourself without relying on expensive or potentially harmful drugs or other medications.

CHAPTER 9

A HISTORICAL OVERVIEW OF NATURAL PRODUCTS IN FOOD

CONTENTS

A natural product, in the broadest sense, is anything derived from life. Other naturally occurring substances once found in living organisms (for example, soil and coal) are also included (e.g. soil, coal). Under a stricter definition, organic material produced by a living species is considered a natural product (Shockley & Dossey, 2014). To begin, the study of natural products resulted in the development of synthetic organic chemistry and semi-synthetic organic chemistry, the latter of which involves modifying the properties of natural products to improve or alter them.

The majority of early drugs were improved through clinical, pharmacological, and chemical research. Salicin, derived from the willow tree Salix Alba, is one of the most well-known anti-inflammatory medications. Morphine, discovered in 1803, is one of several alkaloids found in the *Papaver somniferum* (Opium poppy) plant. In the 1870s, it was discovered that morphine (heroin) could be easily converted to codeine (pain reliever) by heating it in acetic anhydride (painkiller). Even though the Sumerians and Ancient Greeks used opium medicinally, the Arabs considered it addictive. Although *Digitalis purpurea* L. was discovered in Europe in the tenth century, it wasn't until the 1700s that the active ingredient, digitoxin, was discovered to improve cardiac contractility by accelerating cardiac conduction (Saberi *et al.,* 2017). The medication "digitoxin" and its analogs, which have long been used to treat congestive heart failure, are being phased out due to the possibility of long-term side effects. The Food and Drug Administration approved quinine, an antimalarial drug, for sale in the United States in 2004. Malaria, fever, dyspepsia, pharyngitis, and cancer treatment have been a long-standing tradition for thousands of years.

When the British began cultivating the shrub internationally in the mid-nineteenth century, the bark of the shrub was formally used to treat malaria. Pilocarpine, discovered in Pilocarpus jaborandi, is used to treat both chronic open-angle glaucoma and angle-closure glaucoma. In 1994, the FDA approved a pilocarpine oral formulation for the treatment of dry mouth associated with radiation therapy for head and neck cancer. It was also used to stimulate sweat glands so that salt and chloride concentrations could be measured. Sjogren's syndrome, an autoimmune disorder, causes inflammation of the salivary and lacrimal glands. The FDA approved the oral formulation for the treatment of Sjogren's syndrome in 1998.

Natural products have a diverse range of structural characteristics and pharmacological or biological activity because natural selection and evolutionary processes have shaped their value over hundreds of thousands of years. In reality, synthetic organic chemists are unable to match natural molecules' structural diversity. As a result, natural remedies have been used to treat a variety of ailments in both traditional and modern medicine. In pharmaceutical research, synthetic modifications are frequently incorporated into natural compounds to reduce side effects and improve absorption (Ananda *et al.*, 2017). More than half of all FDA-approved medications in the United States are derived from natural materials. Food additives such as spices and herbs, antibacterial agents, and antioxidants are commonly used to preserve freshness and extend the shelf life of food. Organic natural products are used to make our clothing, plastics and rubber, health and beauty products, and even the energy we use to power our cars.

Natural products are the most reliable source of therapeutic candidates (secondary metabolites). However, their use in drug discovery and development has declined in recent years. Even though combinatorial chemistry has been around for decades, natural products continue to be a great source of new low-molecular-weight lead compounds. Many more useful natural lead compounds are awaiting discovery because only about 10% of the world's biodiversity has been studied for biological activity; the issue is access to this chemical diversity.

Cough, cold, and inflammation-fighting oils derived from *Cupressus sempervirens* (Cypress) and *Commiphora* species (Myrrh) can be found on Mesopotamian cuneiform clay tablets. The Ebers Papyrus, an Egyptian medical record, contains over 700 herbal remedies, including gargles, tablets, infusions, and ointments. Natural product use is mentioned in the Chinese Materia Medica, Shennong Herbal, and Tang Herbal. Dioscorides, a Greek physician, documented the collection, preservation, and use of medicinal plants, while Theophrastus, a Greek philosopher, and natural scientist, experimented with therapeutic herbs (Rochfort, 2005). Many of Europe's medieval monasteries were dedicated to preserving the Greco-Roman tradition, while the Arabs pioneered the use of Middle Eastern plants unknown to the Greco-Roman era. The Arabs were the first to establish private pharmacies as early as the eighth century. Avicenna was a Persian pharmacist who also practiced medicine, philosophy, and poetry.

9.1 MEDICINAL PLANTS IN FOLKLORE

For thousands of years, these natural products have been used for medicinal purposes in traditional medicines, treatments, potions, and oils, with many bioactive natural constituents yet to be discovered. Human experimentation with medicinal plants and their natural products has a long history, which has resulted in the most reliable information on the use of medicinal plants and their natural products. Salvia, a plant genus native to the southwest United States and northwest Mexico, has long been used as a birthing aid by Indian tribes in southern California. Salvia ashes were "fried" on male babies in the belief that they would grow up to be the tribe's strongest and healthiest members, free of respiratory ailments for the rest of their lives.

When it's hot outside, the plant *Alhagi maurorum* Medik produces a sweet, sticky substance. Ayurvedic doctors believe the plant can help with anorexia, constipation, dermatosis, epistaxis, fever, leprosy, and obesity, among other ailments. These sugary substances, colloquially known as "manna," are primarily composed of melezitose, sucrose, and inverted sugar. Israelis also boiled the roots and drank the resulting extract to treat violent diarrhea. The Konkani used it to treat asthma, and the Romans used it to treat nasal polyps (Ribeiro et al., 2019). The root of the plant *Ligusticum scoticum*, which grows in Northern Europe and Eastern North America, was used as a sedative and an aphrodisiac in the Faeroe Islands as a remedy for flatulence. Linnaeus discovered *Atropa belladonna* in Central and Southern Europe, Western Asia, North Africa, North America, and New Zealand, among other places (deadly nightshade). Although it was included in the folk medicine collection due to its toxicity (three berries can kill a child), it was removed because it was deemed too dangerous to handle or experiment with.

9.2 MEDICINAL NATURAL PRODUCTS FROM OTHER SOURCES USED IN FOLKLORE

Charcoal made from the fungus *Piptoporus betulinus*, which grows on the bark of birches, has antibacterial and disinfecting properties. Strips of *P. betulinus* were cut and utilized as corn pads as a prophylactic strategy. The fungus *Agaricus campestris* Linnaeux ex Fries is found in temperate regions of the north and south, as well as the Caribbean (the field mushroom). Folklore claims that *A. campestris* was boiled in milk to treat throat cancer.

Lichens were used as colors as early as the 17th and 18th centuries when they were significantly more valuable than eastern spices. Despite significant folklore evidence of their use, no approved lichen-derived drugs are currently available. For millennia, lichens have been used as fundamental elements in perfume, cosmetics, and medicine. *Usnea dillenius* ex Adanson, for example, was initially used to treat scalp diseases when used as an anti-dandruff shampoo component or to treat uncomfortable eyes in Ireland. Stirton boiled *U. subfloridana* with tobacco and butter, cooled it, and used it as a lotion (Reis et al., 2017). Brown dyes were made from the plant *Parmelia omphalodes* (Linnaeus) Acharius, which may be found all across the British Isles. It was usually sprinkled on one's socks before departing on a cruise to relieve foot soreness. It was also used to treat burns and wounds in Scotland, notably in the Highlands.

Traditional medicine, on the other hand, has few applications in the marine environment. A beverage produced from the red algae *Chondrus crispus* and *Mastocarpus stellatus* was traditionally used to treat colds, sore throats, and chest ailments such as tuberculosis. By boiling the alga in milk or water, it was also used to treat kidney disorders and burns. A three-week fast and three spoonfuls of *Porphyra umbilicalis* (Linnaeus) Kützing juice per day have been demonstrated to aid in the treatment of malignancies such as breast cancer. In the Aran Islands, *P. umbilicalis* was allegedly used to alleviate dyspepsia (Raes *et al.,* 2004). Aside from assisting cows with constipation, it was also boiled and given as a supplement in the spring. Natural products can be classified depending on their role in the body, metabolic activity, or source.

9.3 NATURAL PRODUCT FUNCTION

Natural chemicals are classified into two types: primary metabolites and secondary metabolites. Primary metabolites are those that are essential to the organism's survival (i.e. the organism would die without these metabolites). The primary metabolites (nucleic acid, amino acid, sugar, and fat) found in primary metabolites (primary metabolites) are required for the biosynthesis of large macromolecules (DNA, RNA, proteins, carbs, and lipids). Secondary metabolites, on the other hand, are organic compounds that have an impact on organisms other than those that produced them. Secondary metabolites aren't required for an organism to survive, but they do help it compete with other species.

Primary and secondary metabolites are frequently used by organic chemists to characterize natural substances. Secondary metabolites are commonly defined as natural products in the fields of medicinal chemistry and pharmacognosy, which study and employ natural compounds in medicine (Proksch et al., 2003).

9.4 PRIMARY AND SECONDARY METABOLITES (NATURAL PRODUCTS)

Proteins, lipids, nucleic acids, and carbohydrates are all necessary for life, and primary metabolism creates and degrades them all. The chemicals engaged in these activities are referred to as 'primary metabolites.' The process through which organisms biosynthesize secondary metabolites (natural products) is known as biosynthesis (secondary metabolites). Secondary metabolites may be produced by organisms as a protection mechanism against predators.

When an organism adapts to its environment or defends itself against predators, it may require a defensive mechanism that is not required for growth or reproduction. Secondary metabolites, often known as natural products, are produced by photosynthetic intermediates such as glucose and the Krebs cycle (Pop *et al.*, 2019).

Although there are only a limited number of building blocks, the number of secondary metabolites that may be produced is limitless. Acetyl coenzyme A (acetyl-CoA), shikimic acid, mevalonic acid, and 1-deoxyxylulose-5-phosphate are important building blocks in secondary metabolite production. A wide range of processes are involved in the metabolic pathways in which they participate (e.g., alkylation, decarboxylation, aldol creation, and Claisen and Schiff base production).

9.4.1 Primary Metabolites

Primary metabolites are required for all metabolic actions in life. These cells support cellular activities such as nutrition absorption, energy generation, and growth and development.

Their species represent several phyla, and perhaps entire kingdoms. Carbohydrates, lipids, proteins, and nucleic acids are all primary metabolites, and their precursors may be found in high amounts in the human body (DNA and RNA).

These are polymers made up of repeated smaller monomer units that constitute the polymer's structure. Nucleic acid monomers, such as DNA and RNA, are composed of nucleotide bases, which are the building blocks of proteins and carbohydrates.

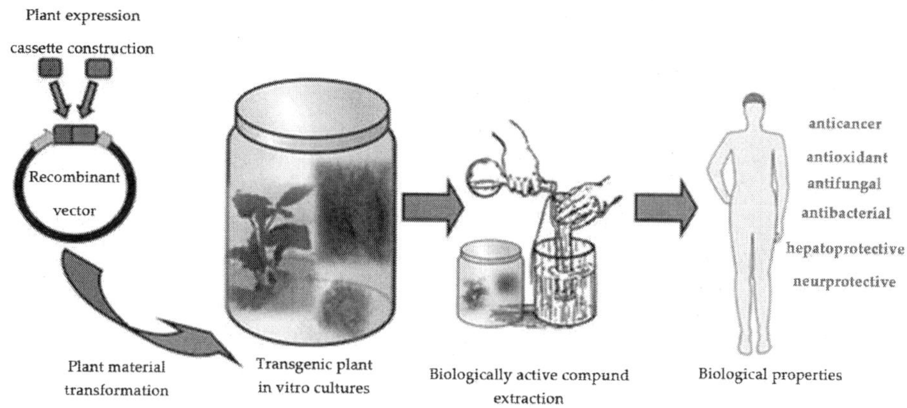

Figure 9.1: Plant metabolites.

(Source: Kowalczyk T, et al., 2020)

Energy production demands the engagement of numerous enzymes. To obtain energy from carbohydrates and lipids, adenosine triphosphate (ATP) molecules are broken down (ATP). Enzymes, which are found in living organisms, operate as catalysts, speeding up chemical processes. Amino acids, the most prevalent kind, are the building blocks of proteins. Basic metabolites are found in cellular and organismal structures (Odhaib *et al.*, 2021). This is seen in membrane components (such as phospholipids) and wall components (such as peptidoglycan and chitin) (proteins). DNA and RNA, the major metabolites of nucleic acids, store and transfer genetic information. Basic metabolites are required for cellular communication, signaling, and transport.

9.4.2 Secondary Metabolites

When it comes to secondary metabolites, primary metabolites take precedence because they are required for life. Secondary metabolites, on the other hand, are frequently limited to a particular species. The deadly nightshade *Atropa belladonna* produces hallucinogenic substances like scopolamine, whereas other plant species do not. This is only the beginning of the discovery of secondary metabolites.

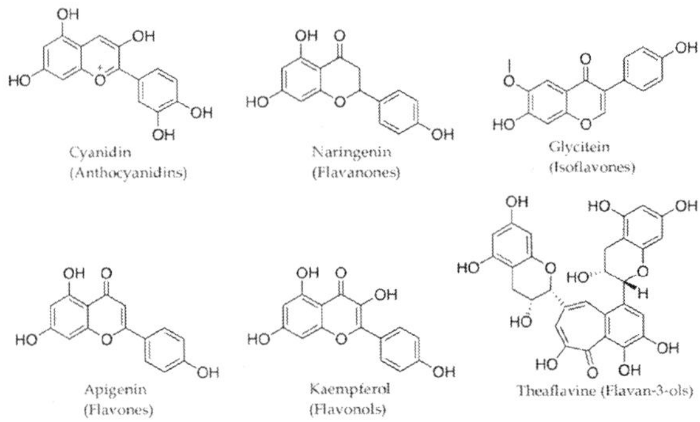

Figure 9.2: Structure of secondary metabolites.

(Source: Yeshi K, Crayn D, et al., 2022)

Secondary metabolites fulfill a variety of purposes. In addition to social signaling molecules, pheromones, which attract and activate symbiotic organisms, siderophores, which deliver nutrients, and competitive weapons (e.g., poisons) used against competitors, prey, and predators are just a few examples. Secondary metabolites that are yet to be found have a range of roles. According to one school of thought, they provide the organism with a competitive edge. Another school of thought holds that, like the immune system, these secondary metabolites have no particular role, but that having the capacity to manufacture these diverse chemical structures is critical. As a result of the organism's long-term exposure, secondary metabolites are produced in small amounts and given more importance.

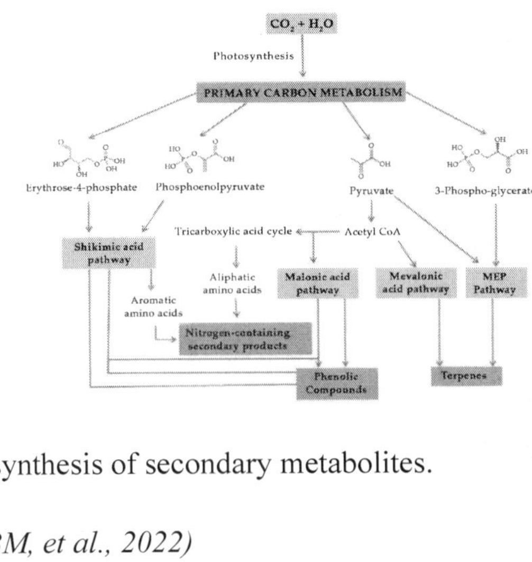

Figure 9.3: Biosynthesis of secondary metabolites.

(Source: Twaij BM, et al., 2022)

Secondary metabolites differ not just inform, but also in the types of molecules, they are composed of. Alkaloids are nitrogen-containing secondary metabolites with an organic structure. They have a plethora of subclasses. Nicotine, the addictive component of tobacco, is used as an example alkaloid. Phenylpropanoids, a chemical compound family, are created by combining phenylalanine and tyrosine.

Cinnamic acid is classified into various subgroups. Phenylpropanoids are volatile taste components of cinnamon. The acetate and malonate building components of polyketides are utilized to generate huge, sophisticated compounds. Aflatoxin B1 is toxic. The fungus Aspergillus produces this polyketide molecule. Fungus-producing Aflatoxin-producing fungus attack stored food crops such as maize and peanuts, contaminating the products (Murdoch et al., 2000). For this reason, aflatoxins are carcinogens (cancer-inducing compounds) (cancer-inducing substances). Cancer of the liver has been related to aflatoxin exposure in food crops. Isoprene-based 5-carbon monomer units make up another significant family of natural compounds, the terpenoids. Terpenoids are present in natural rubber. Isoprene repeating units make up the bulk of it. In the future chapters, we'll dig further into organic structures and look at more instances of these distinct metabolites and how they affect our daily lives.

Where Do We Find Natural Products?

Bacterial, plant, and animal cells, tissues, and secretions can all be used to create natural products. Crude (unfractionated) extracts from any of these sources will produce a diverse range of structurally diverse and frequently novel chemical compounds. Because chemical diversity is derived from biological diversity, many samples from all over the world are used in drug discovery screens and bioassays.

Bioprospecting is the process of looking for natural resources. Understanding the properties of medicinally useful natural substances, also known as pharmacognosy, is critical for those in the pharmaceutical industry. Biological activity in an extract is typically traced back to the source of the extract's composition, which can be a single chemical or a collection of chemically related substances. They can be used in the discovery and development of new medicines, or they can be synthetically modified to improve their biological properties or reduce side effects. New natural chemicals have been discovered using biological sources in the following examples.

9.5 PROKARYOTIC ORGANISMS

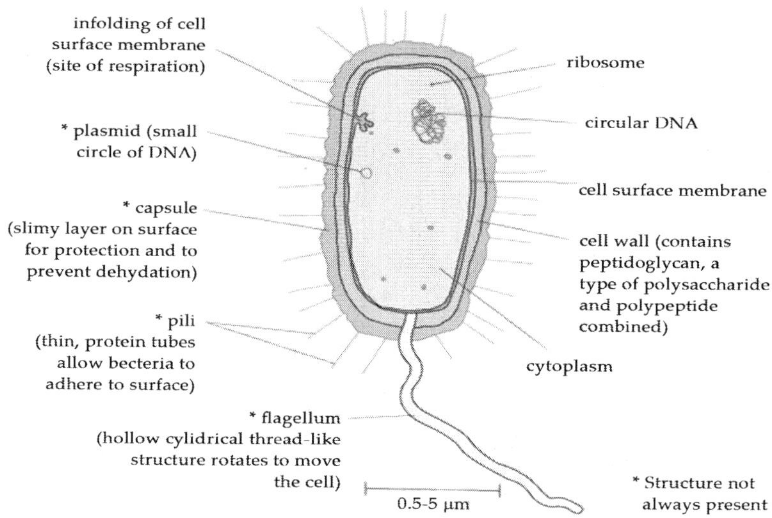

Figure 9.4: Prokaryotic cells.

Prokaryotes are single-celled organisms that lack a membrane. They are devoid of a membrane-bound nucleus, mitochondria, and other organelles. The name of an organism is derived from the Greek words (pro) for "before" and (karyon) for "nut or kernel." Archaea and Bacteria are the two types of prokaryotes found in nature. Animals, plants, fungi, and protozoa all have nuclei and organelles, which belong to the class Eukaryota (Ballester-Sánchez *et al*., 2019).

Water-soluble intracellular components (proteins, DNA, and metabolites) have distinct compartments in prokaryotes, but the cytoplasm, which is surrounded by the cell membrane, does not. Prokaryotic cells are much smaller in size than eukaryotic cells.

9.6 BACTERIA

A typical bacteria is only a few micrometers long and can adopt several shapes, including spheres, rods, and spirals. Bacteria, one of the first living species on the earth, may be found in practically every environment. Microorganisms of many types can be found on the Earth's surface and subsurface.

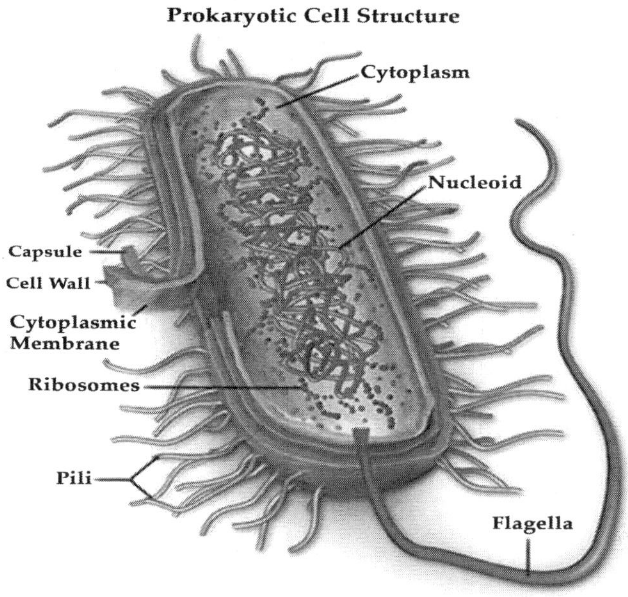

Figure 9.5: Bacterial intracellular structure.

Bacteria have symbiotic and parasitic relationships with plants and animals. Many bacteria remain undiscovered, with cultivable species found in around half of all bacterial phyla. Bacteriology is a field of microbiology that focuses on the study of bacteria. One gram of soil has around 40 million bacterial cells, but a milliliter of clean water contains just one million. Bacteria, in addition to creating natural compounds, are an important source of nutrition (Bacon & Hobson, 2014). Since the discovery of penicillin, many scientists have been looking for environmental bacteria that generate anti-infective natural compounds. Following the collection of soil and water samples from throughout the world, it was determined that *Streptomyces griseus* (the bacterium that makes Streptomycin) is a significant source of antibacterial natural compounds. Amphotericin B, chloramphenicol, and erythromycin (all from Streptomyces species) were produced, as were polymyxin and rifamycins (from *Paenibacillus polymyxa*) and tetracycline (from *Streptomyces* spp) (from *Amycolatopsis rifamycinica*).

While most antibiotics are used to treat infections, some have found their way into other fields of medicine. Botulinum toxin and bleomycin are two antibiotics made from the bacterium *Clostridium botulinum* (derived from *Streptomyces verticillus*). The neurotoxin botulinum toxin causes botulism food poisoning. Botulism is caused by *Clostridium botulinum*, a pathogen that can thrive in improperly sterilized canned meats and other preserved foods. Poisoning can be fatal depending on how much of the toxin is consumed. The eventual result is muscle atrophy and paralysis. This toxin is used cosmetically to minimize the look of wrinkles on the face. It is injected in little amounts into areas such as the forehead to paralyze the muscles that generate wrinkles. Bleomycin is also used to treat Hodgkin's lymphoma, head and neck cancer, and even male testicular cancer (Multari *et al.,* 2015). Metabolic profiling and the isolation of natural chemicals from previously recognized microbes are two recent advances in the field. Secondary metabolites produced by symbionts or endophytes are two examples. Symbionts are little creatures that live close to a larger organism known as a host. Endophytes are non-pathogenic symbionts that cohabit with plants for a portion of their lives. Furthermore, secondary metabolites have become more complicated as a result of the discovery of novel species in tropical settings, bacteria discovered deep below by mining/drilling, and marine bacteria.

9.7 ARCHAEA

Genetic sequencing suggested that an unusual branch of ancient bacterial organisms split off early in the Earth's history. Archaea was uncovered fairly recently in human history, in 1977 by experts. Woese supported separating prokaryotic species into two main divisions, Bacteria and Archaea, based on their genetic differences. Numerous Archaea have developed to live in harsh conditions such as the Polar Regions, hot springs, acidic springs, alkaline springs, salt lakes, and deep ocean water subjected to immense pressure. Extremophiles are Archaea species that can flourish in severe conditions.

Until Woese and Fox proved differently, scientists assumed that prokaryotic extremophiles were bacteria that originated from more common bacterial species. According to studies, they are extraordinarily ancient lifeforms with strong evolutionary ties to Earth's oldest life forms. Woese's finding on Archaea has tremendous ramifications for the quest for extraterrestrial life, as extremophiles may be able to exist in the harsh circumstances seen on other worlds. Because many Archaea adapted to flourish in adverse surroundings, they include enzymes that perform under a broad variety of situations (Lin et al., 2010). These enzymes may be advantageous in biotechnological processes that need high temperatures, pH extremes, high salt concentrations, and/or high pressure, such as those found in the food, chemical, and pharmaceutical sectors.

Pyrococcus furiosus, for example, is an Archaea species that thrives in arid conditions. It is categorized as a hyperthermophile since it lives at significantly greater temperatures than thermophiles want. It is well-known for its optimal growth temperature of 100°C in boiling water (a temperature that would kill most living things) (a temperature that would destroy most living creatures) (a temperature that would destroy most living organisms).

This species was recently identified as a thermostable lactose degrading enzyme. Lactose is a disaccharide sugar contained in milk. Lactose intolerance is a prevalent health issue that causes stomach distress and excessive avoidance of dairy products. Lactose intolerant individuals frequently lack sufficient calcium and vitamin D, as milk is the principal source of these nutrients, which might result in health difficulties. Lactose-free milk production may be a solution to this problem, but it necessitates the use of microbial lactase, which raises the danger of infection. This issue can be remedied by employing thermostable lactase enzymes that are capable of working under pasteurization temperatures. This enzyme functions ideally at 100 degrees Fahrenheit and is thermostable up to 110 degrees Fahrenheit, according to an early study.

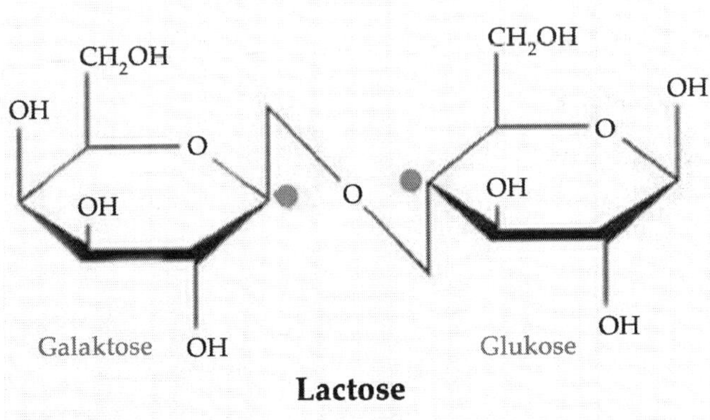

Figure 9.6: Lactose structure.

9.8 EUKARYOTIC ORGANISMS

Protista, Fungi, Plantae, and Animalia are the four eukaryotic kingdoms. Fungi are eukaryotic creatures that are mostly degradative. They might take the shape of a single cell or a swarm of cells. Heterotrophs are creatures that cannot generate nourishment. Plants, for example, are multicellular eukaryotic creatures that can maintain themselves.

Plants, for example, have genuine roots, stalks, and leaves, among other characteristics. Animals are eukaryotic beings that move at least once during their lifetime. All other eukaryotic species that do not belong to the kingdoms Fungi, Plantae, or Animalia are classified as "Protista" (or occasionally Protoctista). Because protists can resemble everything from animals to plants to fungi, this classification is far from optimal(Bis-Souza *et al.*, 2019). Some scientists favor phylogenetic data over traditional protist classification when breaking the kingdom of Protista into smaller groupings of closely related species.

According to Carl Woese's phylogenetic categorization, Protista is divided into three fundamental groups: Ciliates, Flagellates, and Microsporidia. In the next part, we'll look at natural products generated from animals, plants, and fungi. You should also consider the unique natural chemicals created by different protists.

9.9 FUNGI

In heterotrophic eukaryotic animals, fungus absorbs organic substances as their only source of nourishment. Single-celled animals like yeast and molds, as well as multicellular species like mushrooms with fruiting bodies, are among them.

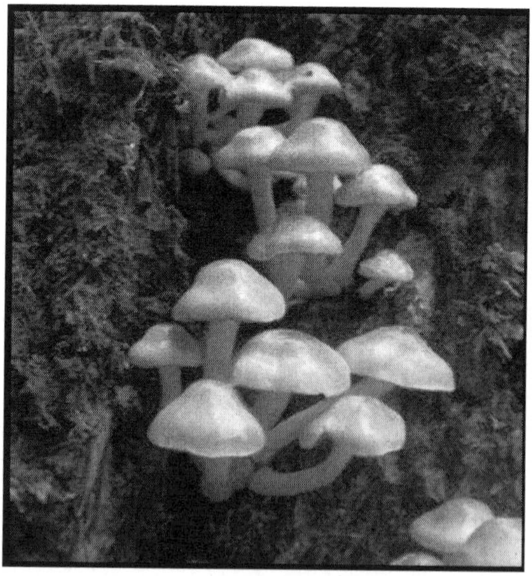

Figure 9.7: Mushrooms that grow in bunches.

A large spectrum of natural byproducts is created by fungus. Death Cap, Destroying Angel, and Fools' Mushroom are just some of the common names given to deadly species. Others have discovered that medications can be incredibly beneficial. Penicillin, cephalosporin (antibacterial medications derived from *Penicillium chrysogenum* and *Cephalosporium acremonium*, respectively), and griseofulvin are only a handful of the numerous antimicrobials made from fungus (an antifungal drug from *Penicillium griseofulvum*)). A fungal metabolite, Lovastatin (made from *Aspergillus terreus*), serves as the predecessor to statins, a class of cholesterol-lowering medications (Bulaj *et al.*, 2016).

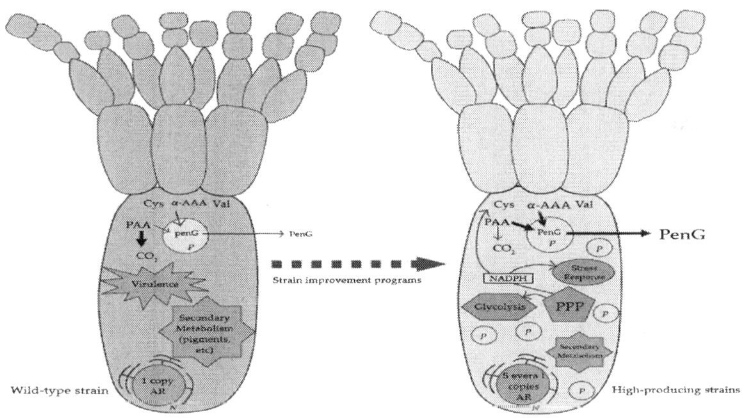

Figure 9.8: Penicillium chrysogenum.

(Source: Barreiro, C., Martín, J. F., et al., 2012)

In the management of postpartum hemorrhage, the vasoconstrictor ergometrine is produced from *Claviceps* spp. Fungus species of the genus Claviceps may commonly be found on cereal crops such as wheat and barley. Human poisoning can occur if considerable quantities of this fungus are ingested after it impacts grain harvests. Convulsions may occur as a result of egotism, or poisoning. Toxic doses of ergometrine might cause gangrene owing to the drug's vasoconstrictive properties. The first areas of the body to be impacted are the fingers and toes, thanks to their lack of vascularization. Peripheral loss of feeling and swelling can develop into edema that finally leads to mortality and tissue loss.

It's hard to think of a fungal byproduct having clinical utility other than cyclosporin. Cyclosporin is an alkaloid cyclic peptide synthesized from amino acid building units. Biologically, this molecule functions as an immunosuppressive agent. Due to its efficacy in preventing organ rejection, it is frequently supplied to patients who have had an organ transplant. The fungus *Tolypocladium inflatum* was the source of cyclosporin, which was identified in 1971. The FDA approved its usage in 1983 following 12 years of laboratory study and clinical testing (Cassani et al., 2020). It is one of the most effective and safe pharmaceuticals essential in a health system, according to the World Health Organization's List of Essential Medicines. *T. inflatum* is an asexual, single-celled form of *Cordyceps subsessilis*, a fungus that also contains a sexually reproducing multicellular life stage. Cyclosporin is synthesized solely during the organism's asexual life stage, showing how an organism's gene expression may fluctuate substantially depending on its life stage or other environmental factors.

9.10 PLANTS

Multicellular eukaryotic animals, such as those found in the plant kingdom, can self-sufficiency and food production. They manufacture all of their food through photosynthesis, a process in which carbon dioxide and water vapor are transformed into simple sugars with the assistance of solar energy. Oxygen is created as a result of this process. To put it another way, plants are a significant supplier of oxygen on a global scale. There are between 250,000 and 300,000 distinct plant species known to exist around the globe. Plants, in addition to producing oxygen and food, are a key source of complex and structurally varied secondary metabolites. This structural variation evolved as a result of natural selection favoring organisms capable of manufacturing anti-herbivory chemicals (feeding deterrents). Even though just a few plants have been thoroughly investigated, pharmacologically active natural compounds have been found and are currently being employed as medicinal agents (Linares *et al.,* 2017). Paclitaxel and vinblastine are anticancer drugs derived from *Taxus brevifolia* and *Catharanthus roseus*, respectively; artemisinin is an antimalarial drug derived from *Artemisia annua*; morphine is an opioid analgesic derived from *Papaver somniferum*, and galantamine is an anticancer drug derived from *Taxus brevifolia* (derived from *Galanthus* spp.).

For thousands of years, medicinal plants have been utilized. Secondary metabolites generated by these species have developed over millions of years to be structurally varied and distinct from those produced by bacteria, insects, fungi, and weather. Their ethnopharmacological qualities were extensively employed as a key source of pharmaceuticals throughout the early stages of drug discovery. According to the WHO, 80 percent of people still use plant-based traditional medicines, and 82 percent of the 122 plant-derived pharmaceuticals are used ethnopharmacological. As people become more aware of the advantages of complementary and alternative medicine, more research into medicinal plants as possible medications is being done, resulting in the discovery of some natural compounds that have since gone on to become well-known pharmaceuticals. Paclitaxel is the most often used medication for breast cancer patients. It is made from the bark of *Taxus brevifolia*. The USDA first gathered the bark in 1962 as part of a National Cancer Institute (NCI) plant screening research. Because a treatment course may require 2 grams of the medication, the bark of three mature 100-year-old trees must generate 1 gram of the medication. The current need is 100–200 kg per year, which is generated in a laboratory. The FDA awarded Taxol its initial approval in 1992 for a variety of purposes. Taxol traces can be found in nature, but it has been synthesized (albeit it is difficult and costly). Baccatin III, which is present in *T. brevifolia* needles and derivatives, may be successfully converted into a structural counterpart.

9.11 ANIMALS

Eukaryotic organisms with more than one cell make up the kingdom Animalia, which includes animals. Heterotrophic animals are mobile at some point in their lives, as previously stated. Vertebrates and invertebrates are the two main groups of animals. Approximately 5 percent of all known animal species are vertebrates, which are animals with a backbone or spine (vertebral column) (vertebral column). Among them are fish, amphibians, reptiles, birds, and mammals. It is only because they lack a backbone that invertebrates have managed to survive. The mollusks, arthropods, annelids (leeches), nematodes (filarial worms, hookworms), flatworms (tapeworms, liver flukes), and cnidarians (clams, oysters, octopus, squid, and snails) are all included in this category (jellyfish) (jellyfish). The science of zoology is concerned with animals.

Bioactive chemicals can also be found naturally in animals (López *et al.*, 2019). Spiders, scorpions, caterpillars, beetle larvae, bees, wasps, centipedes, ants, and frogs have all been given considerable attention in the past few weeks. A macromolecular target in the body is the primary target of venom components (peptides, enzymes, nucleotides lipids, and biogenic amines, for example) (peptides, enzymes, nucleotides lipids, and biogenic amines, for example). Natural selection favors organisms with the ability to kill or paralyze their prey and/or defend themselves against predators, similar to plant feeding deterrents. These organisms have a better chance of survival and reproduction. Chlorotoxin only adheres to brain cancer cells in humans, which is surprising. Gliomas are tumors of the brain or spinal cord that originate in these regions. As a result, it's more likely to develop cancer, a term used to describe cancers with a poor prognosis and a tendency to spread to other organs. Chlorotoxin binds to tumor cells, but not to normal brain tissue. This is surprising. New cancer treatments, diagnostics, and removal procedures have been developed as a result of this property. Phase II clinical trials for TM-601, a synthetic chlorotoxin, are currently underway. Iodine-131 radiotherapy can be used to treat malignant glioma in combination with TM-601. While healthy tissue is protected, malignant brain tumor cells are targeted by TM-601's ability to penetrate the blood-brain barrier and adhere to them. In combination with radioactive Iodine-131, the iodine is drawn to the tumor and preferentially destroys tumor cells.

Toxin derivative BLZ-100, developed by Fred Hutchinson Cancer Research Center scientists and paired with brilliant dye, was also developed. As a result, a steady signal is generated, making the tumor glow as if it were completely painted. When determining the tumor's borders or how far it has grown, this tool can be used in real-time to assist surgeons. In animal studies, this "tumor paint" was found to be effective in treating a wide variety of cancers. When the tumor was taken out of a dog with breast cancer, the surgeons were aware of the huge area in the bottom right that was cancerous, but that was about all they could tell from the clinical examination and previous scans (Karioti et al., 2015). Tumor paint was administered to this dog the day before surgery, allowing the surgeons to see the tumor in the right panel. It was possible to see not only the primary tumor but also previously unnoticed malignant regions.

Aside from meat and dairy products, the bulk of natural food is made up of plant cell fragments. Human small intestine enzymes can't break down these plant cell wall residues. The majority of these residues are made up of cellulose, hemicelluloses, pectic polysaccharides (galacturonic, rhamnogalacturonans), and lignin. Digestion is impeded by the presence of dietary fiber (DF) (DF). Fibrous or not, the term "dietary fiber" has nothing to do with a food's physical characteristics. Chemically or physically, the components of DF have no chemical structure in common apart from the fact that they cannot be digested by enzymes found in the human stomach or small intestine. Soluble dietary fiber (SDF) is distinguished from insoluble dietary fiber (IDF), which is the fiber that is insoluble in water or that precipitates in 78 percent ethanol (that which is soluble in 78 percent ethanol) (that which is soluble in 78 percent ethanol). It's the sum of both insoluble and soluble dietary fiber that makes up total fiber intake (TDF).

There is no consensus on what constitutes dietary fiber (DF), even though the preceding paragraph provided a basic definition of dietary fiber. Many governments and non-profit organizations around the world have adopted and accepted a variety of definitions. It is impossible to give a single explanation for DF's various forms, which include nondigestible and nonabsorbable carbohydrates as well as other chemicals with varying effects on human health. To accurately measure the amount of DF, an official definition of what constitutes DF is needed by various government agencies and the European Union. Everything in the definition has to be quantified in some way, which complicates the definition writing process. There must be two components to any definition of DF, as well. Dietitians need to keep in mind the physiological effects that all DF substances have. If it provides the physiological benefits associated with dietary fiber when consumed, then it is unquestionably dietary fiber. Chemists must first identify all substances capable of producing desired physiological effects to develop methods for determining them; in other words, any definition of DF must allow quantitative measurement for labeling purposes (Khorram & Ramezanian, 2021). It is only known that the molecules in DF are not digested or absorbed and processed in the stomach and that it has a positive impact on health that we can attribute to DF's existence. Because DF is made up of a variety of different nondigestible and nonabsorbable carbohydrates and other substances, it's difficult to come up with a precise definition on which everyone can agree because the difficulty in coming up with a definition that encompasses everything that DF is.

Aside from resistant starch, all hydrocolloids, resistant starch, and naturally occurring polysaccharides such as cellulose (hemicelluloses), pectin (cellulose), and hemi glucose (hemicellulose) are DF components. Because oligosaccharides are indigestible to humans, DF is made entirely of them (that is, all oligosaccharides other than lactose, sucrose, and oligosaccharides generated from starch [that is, maltodextrins]) (that is, all oligosaccharides other than lactose, sucrose, and oligosaccharides generated from starch [that is, maltodextrins]).

A succinct definition of DF has been provided by AACC International. When it comes to the term "dietary fiber," refers to "edible parts of plants and comparable carbohydrates that resist human digestion and absorption, and ferment completely or partially in the large intestine." Dietary fiber consists of polysaccharides, oligosaccharides, lignin, and other plant components. The fiber in the diet can help with constipation, lower cholesterol, and even lower blood sugar levels. All non-starch polysaccharides, whether soluble or insoluble in water, are included in the list of DF components in plant cell walls, including cellulose and lignin. According to the definition's footnote, analogous carbohydrates are carbohydrate-based substances that are not digested or absorbed in the small intestine but are nevertheless not naturally occurring substances in the human body. Maltitol is a carbohydrate substitute according to this definition. Human small intestine digestion is not required for any of the DF components (Karthika & Sureshkumar, 2021). Aside from fruits and vegetables, some low-molecular-weight carbohydrates and hydrocolloids added to processed foods alter their rheological properties and/or provide other functionalities that contribute to total dietary fiber (TDF). Both quantitative and subjectively, each TDF source or component has a distinct physiological effect.

Carbohydrate chemistry can be directly linked to dietary fiber by measuring dietary fiber. For two reasons, a quantitative analysis is critical. Nutritional labeling requires the amount of DF in the serving size of an item. Another reason is that it is legal to estimate a food's caloric content by subtracting insoluble DF from the total carbohydrate value before adding calories from carbohydrate, fat, and protein. The best way to figure out how much DF is in a dish is up for debate. Nutritional labeling requires the use of chemical methods, which is why the ideal method would be one based on physiological responses to meals. A tiny quantity of active vitamin D components is found in most natural diets. Supplementing the diet of persons who lack enough vitamin D can provide a copious supply of 7-Dehydrocholesterol (provitamin D3) and ergosterol (provitamin D2). Provitamins can be found in a range of animal and plant foods, including fish, eggs, yeast, liver, and milk. Ergosterol can only enter the food chain if it is contaminated with fungus. As a result, mushrooms, particularly those found in the wild, contain a high ergosterol concentration. A shortage of vitamin D in animal-based diets might be an issue. It's scarce in meat and dairy products, but plentiful in eggs, fish, and fish oil. Metal traces can be found in plants and vegetable oils (less than 2 percent of the minimum daily requirement).

The Association of Official Analytical Chemists and/or AACC International has developed, validated, and accepted approximately twenty

DF techniques as official methods. Modern DF analytical methods are applied to the data following the general outline. Dry the lipid after it has been extracted with an organic solvent. Heated water is a simple and effective method for gelatinizing starch granules (for example, 95°C for 35 minutes). A thermostable -amylase, a protease, and a glucoamylase should be used sequentially to remove starch and protein. The insoluble residue must be collected and washed. Add ethanol to the soluble fraction to precipitate soluble polysaccharides. Dry, weigh, and process the IDF and SDF fractions. The IDF and SDF values are multiplied to arrive at the TDF. To make TDF, the IDF and SDF fractions are combined after being digested with the three enzymes, and ethanol is added to the dried, weighed, and ashed products (Caporgno & Mathys, 2018).

When four liters of 95 percent ethanol are added, the digestion products that are absorbed but not precipitated are not included in this method, which is the only significant drawback (for example, low-molecular-weight components of fructooligosaccharides [FOS]) (for example, low-molecular-weight components of fructooligosaccharides [FOS]). Such soluble components in the soluble fraction can be identified using HPLC (high-performance liquid chromatography) (high-performance liquid chromatography). Vitamin D is present in most natural diets in a small amount. 7-Dehydrocholesterol (provitamin D3) and ergosterol (provitamin D2) are abundant in animals and plants, respectively, and can provide humans' diets with adequate vitamin D. Provitamins are found in fish, eggs, yeast, liver, milk, and some vegetables, such as cabbage. To some, fungal contamination is the only way ergosterol enters the food chain. A lot of ergosterol can be found in mushrooms that are found in the wild.

Vitamin D deficiency is common in foods derived from animals that have not been fortified. Eggs, fish, and fish liver oils contain significant amounts, while meat and dairy products contain far less. Botanical sources of the element include plants and vegetable oils, both of which contain negligible amounts of it.

9.12 NATURALLY OCCURRING TOXINS IN PLANT-BASED FOODS

Over two-thirds of the world's 300,000 plant species are toxic. When foraging for edibles such as wild mushrooms, berries, and other plants, poisoning is prevalent. There are just a few hundred plant species consumed daily across the world, yet many of them may be detrimental to the human body if taken in high numbers or if not properly prepared before consumption. Plant parts that are edible or toxic vary by species; edible portions include things like leaves and buds, while dangerous parts include things like roots and tubers. Toxins that are similar or dissimilar in plants of the same species are not rare. These variables influence a plant's poisonous content and dispersion as it grows in diverse conditions.

Plant components such as flowers and seeds are high in defensive chemicals. These chemicals may be created or maintained more quickly in potato sprouts during critical phases of growth, such as buds, seedlings, or immature tissue (Karwowska *et al.*, 2021). Natural poisons are found in a variety of food plants, including glycoalkaloids in potatoes, cyanide-producing compounds in bitter apricot seeds, and enzyme inhibitors and lectins in soya beans and other legumes.

9.13 TOXIC NATURAL TOXINS IN HUMAN FOOD

Natural poisons may be derived from animal metabolic products or compounds that migrate up the food chain. Even though terrestrial animal poisoning is uncommon, marine poisons are a common cause of poisoning in many parts of the world. Toxic microalgae in the water produce marine poisons, which are consumed by sea organisms such as mussels, crabs, and fish. Tetrodotoxin, a marine neurotoxin, has been linked to several microorganisms. It is carried by over 90 species of pufferfish, and even a little quantity can be fatal. Ciguatoxin, a toxin found in over 300 different species, is toxic to coral reef fish and can cause seafood poisoning in humans. Another type of seafood poisoning is histamine, which is produced when bacteria break down scombroid fish. The world is home to over 1,200 different types of poisonous and venomous animals. Even if the majority of these hazardous glands or tissue are not eaten, they must be avoided. The gallbladder of grass carp, for example, contains Cuprinol-related compounds that can cause food poisoning although they are not lethal or hazardous when consumed (Kau *et al.,* 2011).

9.14 FOOD POISONING'S DANGERS

Natural poisons included in food can produce a wide range of clinical symptoms as well as short- and long-term health consequences. Acute symptoms might range from abdominal discomfort to neurological disorders, breathing difficulty to death. Children and the elderly, as well as other marginalized groups, are particularly vulnerable. Many marine toxins found in mussels and other seafood can cause serious health problems in just hours or minutes. If uncooked mushrooms and plants, such as ginkgo seeds and bitter apricot seeds, are consumed, they can cause severe poisoning. Plant poisoning, such as the numerous alkaloids found in many plants, is more likely to cause chronic toxicity. Large amounts of pyrrolizidine alkaloids, which are abundant in plants such as weeds and crops, can harm the liver. The amount of food required to cause poisoning is determined by the toxin concentration and the individual's sensitivity.

9.15 STRATEGIES FOR MITIGATING THE EFFECTS OF POTENTIAL RISKS

By using appropriate food processing methods, such as thorough cooking, it is possible to eliminate or greatly reduce the toxic content of food. If the toxin cannot be reduced or removed, consumption should be restricted. Beans are thoroughly cooked to remove enzyme inhibitors and lectins. Some of the cyanide-producing components in food can be removed by soaking or boiling it. Toxins are removed from tissue using organs such as the skin and gonad of some fish (Dayan et al., 2009). Because the body is capable of detoxifying small amounts of many potentially harmful treatments, the toxicity of a drug is determined by its concentration, the amount consumed, and the individual's health. As a general rule, people should use safe food processing methods and eat a varied and balanced diet to reduce their exposure to natural contaminants. To sum up, we believe that combining metabolomics and natural product discovery techniques would be beneficial on several different levels. Increased identifications in our metabolomics data can help us start by providing novel structures for testing bioactivity in any condition under investigation. Chemical characterization operations on diverse natural resource species can also be accelerated and increased throughput by employing metabolomics technology in parallel. For the second time, chemists working with natural products have amassed libraries of active and inert pure chemicals that can now be analyzed to generate mass spectral and NMR spectral libraries, improving the biological interpretation of metabolomics data. To advance natural product chemistry discovery, smaller molecule compounds that are detectable in biological systems (i.e., primary and secondary metabolites) have been able to be detected thanks to advances in analytical instrumentation and sophisticated hyphenation of separation techniques with highly sensitive detectors.

CHAPTER 10

THE ROLE OF NATURAL PRODUCTS IN MODERN DRUG DISCOVERY

CONTENTS

10.1: INTRODUCTION

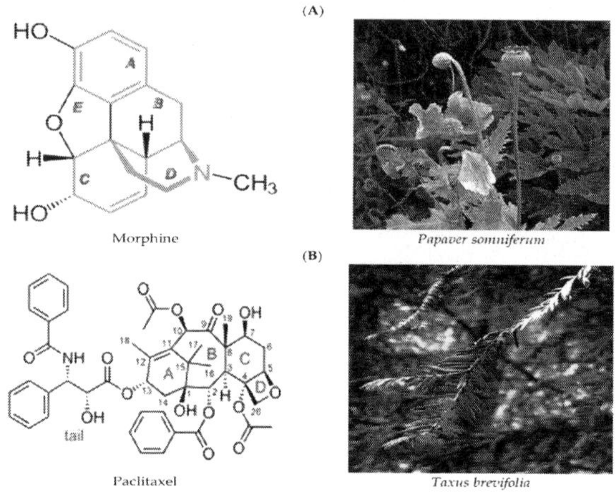

Figure 10.1. The role of natural products in drug discovery.

(Source: Thomford NE, Senthebane DA, et, al., 2018)

Since immemorial natural products such as plants, animal products, and minerals have contributed to the treatment of various illnesses. In the past, people relied on these products to produce medicinal products that were used to treat various diseases. There is evidence that plants, animals, and minerals were used to make medicine that was used by locals. It is vital to note that other microorganisms were used to make medicine and the practice continued for many centuries. These organic substances and chemicals have been extensively indicated for the management of a broad range of disorders. Since at least 4,000 years ago, the poppy, as well as the marijuana plant, have both been utilized medicinally. When Friedrich Serturner discovered the alkaloid morphine inside the poppy in 1806, he spurred the quest for alternative plant-derived medications (Da Silva et al., 2016). Also derived from poppy, Pierre-Jean Robiquet discovered the anti-tussive substance codeine in 1824, and George Merck Fraz discovered the anti-spasmodic alkaloid papaverine in 1848, all of which were discovered by the same plant. Some of the many active principles discovered in plants include atropine, which Mein discovered in 1831 from Atropos bellidonii; caffeine, found by Runge in 1820 in the coffee plant Coffea arabica; digoxin in 1869 by Claude-Adolphe Nativelle in Digitalis lanata; and curare in 1943 by the Germans Winsterstein and Dutchers in the South American plant Chondrodendron tomentosum.

As a result of the inability of other clinical research methodologies, there seems to be a surge in the number of people interested in organic product studies. This is because natural products can be used to make medicines that can help people with illnesses such as immunosuppressive drugs, infections, and metabolic disorders, among other things. Organic product studies constantly look at a range of lead designs that might be exploited by healthcare companies to generate novel medications. Organic products are and will continue to be major sources of novel pharmaceutical ingredients, there can be no question about that. However, although organic products have historically performed a vital effect on drug development, the majority of Big Pharma firms have either canceled or significantly downsized existing organic product activities in recent years (Dixon & Sumner, 2003). Over the previous few years, there has been an increment in the number of natural products used in pharmaceuticals that have been named among the top-selling ethical medications in the universe. It took a long time to identify new drugs from natural products because of the several rounds of separating and structural elucidation that were necessary. Advances in novel therapeutic elucidation, as well as lead structure identification, are likely to contribute to new techniques to enhance and speed up the combined medicinal chemistry process. The development of novel medicines is being revolutionized by technological advances that include mechanized separation processes, elevated screening, as well as combinatorial chemistry.

10.2: HOW PLANTS AND NATURE ACT AS SOURCES OF DRUG COMPOUNDS

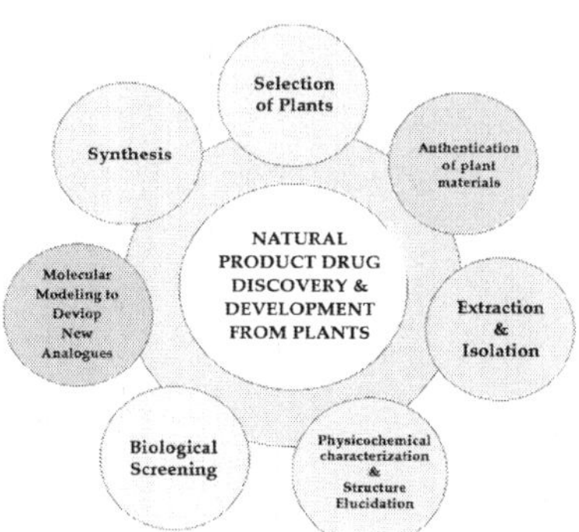

Figure 10.2: Plants as natural sources of drug compounds.

(Source: Najmi A, Javed SA, et al., 2022)

Pharma study has relied heavily on natural sources since many medications are derived from natural materials. Furthermore, it is believed that 40 percent of all medications are all either organic compounds or chemically synthesized derivatives of natural compounds. Research on these ancient remedies, which were mostly obtained from nature, became the foundation of many of the first drugs which include aspirin, digitoxin, quinine, as well as pilocarpine. Many novel clinical prospects and medications are still being discovered by using organic remedies despite opposition from other approaches to drug development. Mostly in anticancer, hypertensive medication, anti-infective, immunosuppressive, and neurological illness treatment domains, these substances were already a substantial source of novel medications, and several of them have subsequently gone more into medical studies or entered the market (Kadam & Prabhasankar, 2010). As a result, a natural product-derived medications are not only a reliable form of drug leads as well as a substantial source of revenue for several firms. Organic product studies constantly look at a range of lead structures that might be exploited by healthcare companies to generate novel medications. These authorized molecules, which span a broad range of chemical biodiversity, highlight the value of bioactive components in current drug development efforts.

The primary contributor of biologically active compounds has been organic compounds, which have more structural variety than synthesized molecules, and will continue to play a vital role in the discovery of novel medications. As a result of biological activity-directed isolation approaches, several valuable medications have been discovered from herbal medicines. In the course of this investigation, the role of earth's resources in the medical arsenal was thoroughly examined. Medical research and development may benefit from the usage of natural products, which are chemical compounds or substances created by living organisms and found in the environment. Even though this substance can be made through complete synthesizing, it is still a commodity. This might be derived using terrestrial plants, sea creatures, or microbe fermenting broths. Many of these sources often yield an extract that is full of unique, structurally distinct chemical components (Jacob *et al.*, 2020). Several organic products are too complicated and costly to synthesize on a mass scale since not all naturally occurring substances can be entirely synthesized. Penicillin, morphine, as well as paclitaxel, were all examples of this class of medication. The only way to get these substances is to extract them from their natural origin, a procedure that may be time-consuming, costly, and even dangerous. Additionally, gathering yields only a restricted variety of structural counterparts. Additional issues include the fact that isolated natural chemicals typically perform differently than their original counterparts due to synergy and the possibility of combining, for example, antibacterial substances alongside compounds that activate diverse body's immune pathways.

Advanced plant metabolites have a wide range of diverse biological functions. Only a very small percentage of chemotherapeutics now utilized in the industrialized world has already been synthesized using this method. Some, like taxol as well as vincristine, were challenging to manufacture *in vitro* because of their structural complexity. Several unnatural, synthetic medications have adverse reactions that were only accepted as therapies for grave illnesses like cancer. Compounds from therapeutic medicinal and aromatic plant items might escape the adverse effects of manufactured medications since they must increase in live cells. The use of semi-synthetic techniques may be able to alleviate some of these issues. The biochemical intermediary, instead of the ultimate lead chemical, is frequently harvested again from its natural origin in this manner (Ibrahim *et al.*, 2015). Conventional synthesis might then be used to transform the intermediary into the finished piece. Both benefits and disadvantages may be derived from this strategy. In the first place, the intermediary is more readily retrieved than the final deliverable itself. Moreover, it could make it possible to synthesize analogs of the ultimate item. An example of this method is the use of semi-penicillins. It was recently discovered that 10-deacetylbaccatin may be synthesized from the yew needles using a four-stage process. Pharma companies are now again paying attention to natural product-based drug development because of new technology innovations that offer better financial results, such as synthetic peptides.

For millennia, humans have been linked to the natural world, especially microorganisms and vegetative substances in their original environment. In the search for novel drug-discovery bioactive molecules, they have been critical tools. In addition, organic drugs provided as leads might be refined by synthesis techniques. Antimicrobials, antitumors, diuretics, and anti-inflammatory medications, for example, accounted for an even larger percentage of all authorized small molecules that were created from naturally occurring chemical entities. In addition, the latter is acknowledged as a significant repository of biological variety. Because fewer natural compounds with therapeutic characteristics are available as a consequence of extinction in the animal kingdom, medical science may have fewer options for treating sickness. Selecting as well as evaluating natural compounds for pharmaceutical research as potential therapeutics was covered in depth. Most of these organic products have also been claimed to have contributed to the invention of new medications.

10.3 HOW HAVE NATURAL PRODUCTS SUCCEEDED IN MODERN DRUG DISCOVERY?

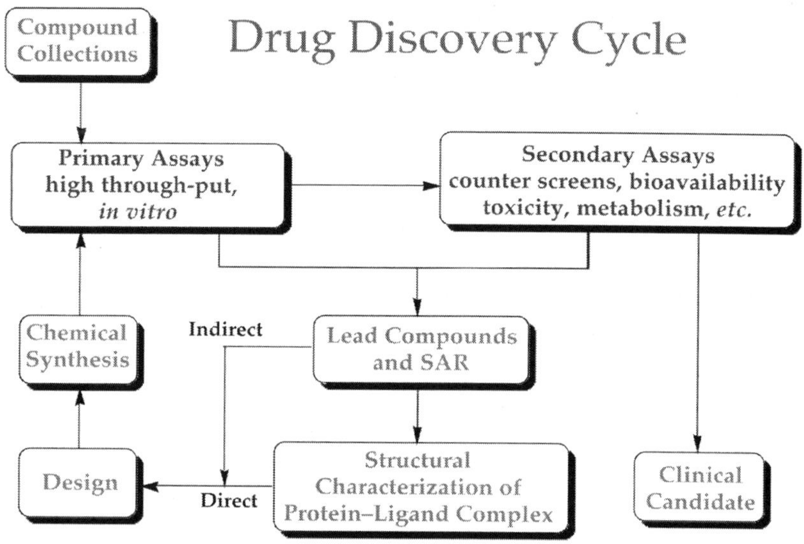

Figure 10.3: How drugs are derived from natural products.

With an integrated strategy that includes many research technologies and the emerging field of "integrative biology," the search for novel plant-derived drugs is bound to be a breakthrough. To find novel, reliable, and cost-effective medicines, herbal compounds will continue to play an important role. Organic product drug development projects need a paradigm shift in the medical firm's thinking and resources. When it comes to drug-related properties, natural items can't be beaten by synthetics. Organic substances have a very wide range of molecular and anatomical variations. Biological evolution is some other major benefit of organic products. The biosynthetic pathway of natural consumer products requires frequent interactions with enzymatic modulators, and binding to other peptides is a common physiological role for several organic compounds (Hou & Xu, 2022). Because natural compounds may react with several other compounds, which is an essential step in the process of creating an effective medicine, this capacity might be regarded scientifically confirmed. Many natural compounds have enhanced binding properties compared to synthetic substances, which is an expected but sometimes neglected feature. Natural products' more complicated steric structure is most likely a factor.

Aside from that, natural compounds have relatively high molecular masses than synthetically produced ones. Analytical chemistry plays a role in the development of natural products because they allow researchers to take advantage of the wide range of chemical compositions and biologically active compounds that these items possess. Different substrates and computerized synthesis of novel chemical compounds for psychotropic assessment will be aided by the examination of structured chemical databases that include a broad range of chemotypes as well as information on potential target genomic sequences. Some 50% of all prescription pharmaceuticals in developed countries are derived or manufactured from natural compounds, the only accessible sources of which are animals, oceans, plants, as well as micro-organisms (Haque *et al.*, 2020). As a result of their morphological and physiological variables, terrestrial plants are believed to be a distinct and renewable energy resource for identifying possible novel medications or biochemical substances. That natural products, with their intrinsic large-scale structural diversity, have and will continue to be the primary sources of physiologically relevant compounds is not supported by any data.

Utilizing three factors, you can figure out how significant natural products are in the early diagnosis of diseases in humans. These three factors are the rate at which novel chemical institutions of a wide range of structures are being created, as well as how often these substances are used as layouts for semi-structured and complete alteration. Organic materials are a significant resource in novel pharmaceuticals, and they might even potentially serve as useful lead molecules for more customization even during the creation of new medicines. Natural products have a big role in drug development because of the wide variety of configurations and complicated carbon skeletons found in these substances. Ecological compatibility, as well as drug-like characteristics of the material secondary metabolites, are typically considered superior to those of completely manufactured compounds, making them excellent candidates for therapeutic development.

10.4: WAYS IN WHICH NATURAL PRODUCTS ARE USED TO PRODUCE MODERN DRUGS

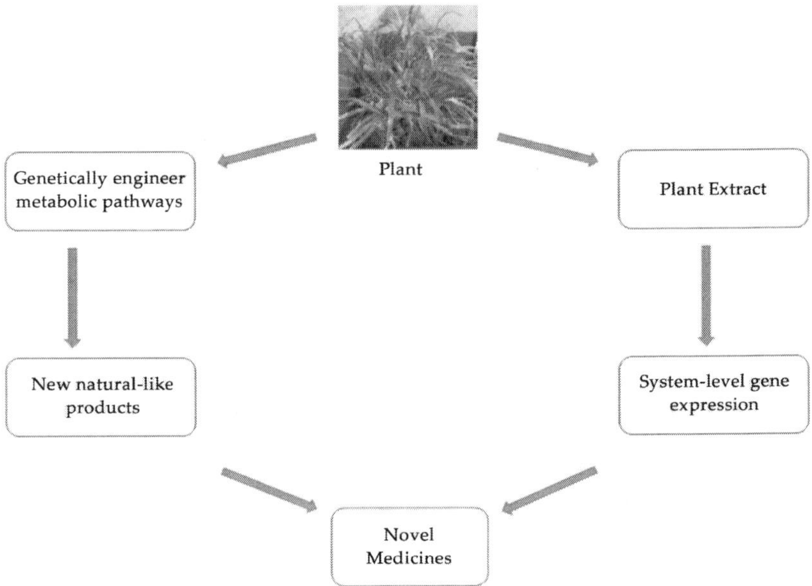

Figure 10.4: Plants as sources of medicine.

(Source: Thomford NE, Senthebane DA, et, al., 2019)

Since biochemical processes, biomedical engineering, and genetics have become more well-understood, drug development has become more time-sensitive. Pharma companies are turning to chemically synthesized analogs because of the emergence of new sequential biotechnological processes and computational approaches, as well as the inability of natural remedies to keep up with rising rivalry for new characters of treatments at a quicker rate. Despite their appreciation and respect for nature's position as the founding father of organic medicine collections, pharma companies are wary of researching this topic. Combination and high-throughput screening (HTS) have failed to generate widely used chemical entities, resulting in a shift in thinking about new techniques.

When extracting and isolating, the old methods were too time-consuming and could not meet the needs of high-tech systems. Every institution that does Natural Product-based Drug Discovery (NPDD) programs uses actinomycetes and fungi as testing materials or practically every institution that does so. Viruses, vegetation, and therapeutic herbs are the next topics covered. Some companies use invertebrates including microalgae to check their products. Insects are seldom used for commercial purposes. Some people, on the other hand, are looking for bacteria from odd habitats. Because natural compounds are seldom released as drugs in their original form, many nations will be discouraged from participating in the pharmaceutical invention process if they have unrealistic aspirations about the return on their investment. Pharmacognosy is the science that gives the techniques for identifying, selecting, and processing natural materials that are intended for medical use. Typically, the plant-derived component seems to have some degree of environmental function, and this molecule is referred to as one of the active components. A composition with this kind of architecture may function as a lead chemical. Many of today's medications are derived straight from plants or other naturally occurring sources.

To develop a novel treatment for a condition, a huge library of compounds is examined for their capacity to alter the target. This approach is called high-throughput screening. HTS may also be used to demonstrate how well a molecule binds to a certain target. Finding a chemical that interferes solely with both the selected target but never with other, connected targets is desirable. Cross-screening is used to determine if the hits on the selected target would conflict with certain other connected targets to accomplish this goal. When a chemical hits many independent receptors during testing, it is even more sufficient to evoke off-target poisoning in the clinical setting. In the early stages of drug discovery, it is quite improbable that a great medication contender will be uncovered. Some molecules are said to have significant action and pharmacophores may be built by looking for common chemical properties across the active molecules. Structure-activity connections will be used by drug design at this stage to enhance certain properties of the lead drug.

These vetting intervals will be repeated many times, so it is anticipated that the characteristics of current biological organizations will get better during this time. The best substances can then be assessed *in vitro* and also in a living animal model to see if they can help with a diagnostic manual of their choice. Although HTS is a frequent strategy for discovering new drugs, there are others. In many cases, it is feasible to start with a compound that inherently is among the necessary characteristics. Alternatively, such a molecule may be derived from a plant origin or even a commercially available medicine that could still be refined. In other cases, machine techniques are applied for filtering, and simulated libraries are "stationed" to a destination to station them. In addition to pharmaceutical research, drug development is a crucial step in the process. In this step, the natural and physiological features of the targeted are investigated, and a forecast is made about the types of molecules that would be able to bind to an active center. Innovative pharmacophores may be discovered extremely quickly as a result of these efforts. After one lead chemical series has already been produced that exhibits appropriate target concentration and exclusivity, as well as desirable drug-like features, one or two molecules will be offered for further exploration as potential drugs. The finest among these will often be referred to it as "chemical entities," whereas others will be referred to as the "backup compound."

Because of sequencing technologies, the needle may be buried in a larger haystack. There is no doubt that natural chemicals have biological effects when they are found. To be successful in organic product studies, you need years of expertise, notably in classification. This expertise will be lost forever if it isn't preserved. Since many highly sophisticated biotech businesses will play a critical role in NPDD, one possibility is to outsource the operation. The latest advances in creative manufacturing, microbial genomics, as well as vetting techniques are causing a renaissance in current plant-derived exploration. Natural compounds' chemical diversity may be used in the building of combinatorial libraries to enhance their intrinsic metabolic processes or substance qualities (Halloran *et al.*, 2015). This may be accomplished by quasi alteration of the original molecule or through completely synthetic approaches when critical structural features essential for bioactive compounds are specified and improved using machine drug design tools. More precise *in vitro* and *in vivo* studies, targeting, and methods are now accessible than in the past. Pharmacological, phytochemistry, microbiological, and single-molecule approaches are all used in contemporary herbal drug exploration. For research at the molecular scale, a fundamental change from the identification of specific bioactive compounds may be used to highlight the multi-constituent backbone of reactive extracts. The danger of biological diversity annihilation owing to climate change and other ecological factors is also quite significant now. As a result, indigenous natural environments must be identified and thoroughly studied to be used in medication development. Ancient treatment as well as the development of new natural products rely on a regular flow of herbal medicines.

Pharmaceuticals must go ahead and capitalize on the understanding that has been accumulated via conventional medical practices and procedures. These latter ideas have the potential to heal a variety of illnesses and problems, but they must first be scientifically validated. Because the border between contemporary and conventional treatments is still hazy, the initial step in focusing study on medicinal herbs is to scientifically evaluate the pharmacological effects of herbal medications (Hathwar et al., 2012). This may make the evaluation of performance simpler if the line between logical and anecdotal treatment is formed having to take into consideration psychodynamic consequences connected with the active chemicals, as well as their normal purposes. Considering firms have begun integrating ancient expertise in the creation of their preparations and drug research initiatives is a heartening trend.

REFERENCES

1. Acosta-Estrada, B. A., Reyes, A., Rosell, C. M., Rodrigo, D., & Ibarra-Herrera, C. C. (2021). Benefits and Challenges in the Incorporation of Insects in Food Products. *Frontiers in Nutrition, 8*.
2. Ambuja, S. R., & Rajakumar, S. N. (2018). Review On "Dietary Fiber Incorporated Dairy Foods: A Healthy Trend". *Int. J. Eng. Res. Appl, 8*, 34-40.
3. Ananda, A. P., Manukumar, H. M., Umesha, S., Soumya, G., Priyanka, D., Mohan Kumar, A. S., & Savitha, K. R. (2017). A relook at food packaging for cost effective by incorporation of novel technologies. *Journal of Packaging Technology and Research, 1*(2), 67-85.
4. Ballester-Sánchez, J., Gil, J. V., Haros, C. M., & Fernández-Espinar, M. T. (2019). Effect of incorporating white, red or black quinoa flours on free and bound polyphenol content, antioxidant activity and colour of bread. *Plant Foods for Human Nutrition, 74*(2), 185-191.
5. Bacon, P., & Hobson, C. (2014). Incorporating natural disasters into the human security agenda. *HOBSON, Christopher; BACON, Paul; CAMERON, Robin, Human security and natural disasters. Routledge, Nueva York, Routledge*, 1-21.
6. Barreiro, C., Martín, J. F., & García-Estrada, C. (2012). Proteomics shows new faces for the old penicillin producer Penicillium chrysogenum. *Journal of biomedicine & biotechnology, 2012*, 105109.
7. Bis-Souza, C. V., Barba, F. J., Lorenzo, J. M., Penna, A. B., & Barretto, A. C. S. (2019). New strategies for the development of innovative fermented meat products: a review regarding the incorporation of probiotics and dietary fibers. *Food Reviews International, 35*(5), 467-484.

8. Bulaj, G., M Ahern, M., Kuhn, A., S Judkins, Z., C Bowen, R., & Chen, Y. (2016). Incorporating natural products, pharmaceutical drugs, self-care and digital/mobile health technologies into molecular-behavioral combination therapies for chronic diseases. *Current clinical pharmacology*, *11*(2), 128-145.

9. Cassani, L., Gomez-Zavaglia, A., Jimenez-Lopez, C., Lourenço-Lopes, C., Prieto, M. A., & Simal-Gandara, J. (2020). Seaweed-based natural ingredients: Stability of phlorotannins during extraction, storage, passage through the gastrointestinal tract and potential incorporation into functional foods. *Food Research International*, *137*, 109676.

10. Caporgno, M. P., & Mathys, A. (2018). Trends in microalgae incorporation into innovative food products with potential health benefits. *Frontiers in nutrition*, *5*, 58.

11. Dayan, F. E., Cantrell, C. L., & Duke, S. O. (2009). Natural products in crop protection. *Bioorganic & medicinal chemistry*, *17*(12), 4022-4034.

12. Da Silva, B. V., Barreira, J. C., & Oliveira, M. B. P. (2016). Natural phytochemicals and probiotics as bioactive ingredients for functional foods: Extraction, biochemistry and protected-delivery technologies. *Trends in Food Science & Technology*, *50*, 144-158.

13. Dai G, Shen Q, Zhang Y, Bian X. Biosynthesis of Fungal Natural Products Involving Two Separate Pathway Crosstalk. *Journal of Fungi*. 2022; 8(3):320.

14. Dixon, R. A., & Sumner, L. W. (2003). Legume natural products: understanding and manipulating complex pathways for human and animal health. *Plant Physiology*, *131*(3), 878-885.

15. Drewnowski A, Maillot M, Papanikolaou Y, Jones JM, Rodriguez J, Slavin J, Angadi SS, Comerford KB. A New Carbohydrate Food Quality Scoring System to Reflect Dietary Guidelines: An Expert Panel Report. *Nutrients*. 2022; 14(7):1485.

16. Fabani, M. P., Luna, L., Baroni, M. V., Monferran, M. V., Ighani, M., Tapia, A.,& Feresin, G. E. (2013). Pistachio (Pistacia vera var Kerman) from Argentinean cultivars. A natural product with potential to improve human health. *Journal of Functional Foods*, *5*(3), 1347-1356.

17. Francesconi, K. A. (2007). Toxic metal species and food regulations—making a healthy choice. *Analyst*, *132*(1), 17-20.

18. Ferreira, C. D., & Nunes, I. L. (2019). Oil nanoencapsulation: development, application, and incorporation into the food market. *Nanoscale research letters*, *14*(1), 1-13.
19. Hathwar, S. C., Rai, A. K., Modi, V. K., & Narayan, B. (2012). Characteristics and consumer acceptance of healthier meat and meat product formulations—a review. *Journal of food science and technology*, *49*(6), 653-664.
20. Halloran, A., Vantomme, P., Hanboonsong, Y., & Ekesi, S. (2015). Regulating edible insects: the challenge of addressing food security, nature conservation, and the erosion of traditional food culture. *Food Security*, *7*(3), 739-746.
21. Haque, A., Ahmad, S., & Khan, I. (2020). Incorporation of Food Materials as a Source of Dietary Fibers and Natural Antioxidants in Meat Products and their Effect on Product Quality and Human Health: A Mini Review. *Journal of Buffalo Science*, *9*, 76-83.
22. Hou, W., & Xu, H. (2022). Incorporating Selenium into Heterocycles and Natural Products— From Chemical Properties to Pharmacological Activities. *Journal of Medicinal Chemistry*, *65*(6), 4436-4456.
23. Ibrahim, U. K., Salleh, R. M., & Maqsood-ul-Haque, S. N. S. (2015). Bread towards functional food: an overview. *International Journal of Food Engineering*, *1*(1), 39-43.
24. Jacob, A., Johnson, K., Cohen, R., & Carlson, S. E. (2020). Incorporating natural ecosystems into global health and food security programmes. *Bulletin of the World Health Organization*, *98*(8), 576.
25. Kadam, S. U., & Prabhasankar, P. (2010). Marine foods as functional ingredients in bakery and pasta products. *Food Research International*, *43*(8), 1975-1980.
26. Kau, A. L., Ahern, P. P., Griffin, N. W., Goodman, A. L., & Gordon, J. I. (2011). Human nutrition, the gut microbiome and the immune system. *Nature*, *474*(7351), 327-336.
27. Karwowska, M., Stadnik, J., Stasiak, D. M., Wójciak, K., & Lorenzo, J. M. (2021). Strategies to improve the nutritional value of meat products: incorporation of bioactive compounds, reduction or elimination of harmful components and alternative technologies. *International Journal of Food Science & Technology*, *56*(12), 6142-6156.

28. Karthika, C., & Sureshkumar, R. (2021). Incorporation of natural assumption to deal with cancer. *Environmental Science and Pollution Research*, *28*(5), 4902-4917.
29. Khorram, F., & Ramezanian, A. (2021). Cinnamon essential oil incorporated in shellac, a novel bio-product to maintain quality of 'Thomson navel'orange fruit. *Journal of Food Science and Technology*, *58*(8), 2963-2972.
30. Kowalczyk T, Wieczfinska J, Skała E, Śliwiński T, Sitarek P. Transgenesis as a Tool for the Efficient Production of Selected Secondary Metabolites from Plant *in vitro* Cultures. *Plants*. 2020; 9(2):132.
31. Karioti, A., Ceruso, M., Carta, F., Bilia, A. R., & Supuran, C. T. (2015). New natural product carbonic anhydrase inhibitors incorporating phenol moieties. *Bioorganic & Medicinal Chemistry*, *23*(22), 7219-7225.
32. Kwan DH, Schulz F. The Stereochemistry of Complex Polyketide Biosynthesis by Modular Polyketide Synthases. *Molecules*. 2011; 16(7):6092-6115.
33. López, C. J., Caleja, C., Prieto, M. A., Sokovic, M., Calhelha, R. C., Barros, L., & Ferreira, I. C. (2019). Stability of a cyanidin-3-O-glucoside extract obtained from Arbutus unedo L. and incorporation into wafers for colouring purposes. *Food chemistry*, *275*, 426-438.
34. Linares, D. M., Gómez, C., Renes, E., Fresno, J. M., Tornadijo, M. E., Ross, R. P., & Stanton, C. (2017). Lactic acid bacteria and bifidobacteria with potential to design natural biofunctional health-promoting dairy foods. *Frontiers in microbiology*, *8*, 846.
35. Lin, X., Racette, S. B., Lefevre, M., Spearie, C. A., Most, M., Ma, L., & Ostlund, R. E. (2010). The effects of phytosterols present in natural food matrices on cholesterol metabolism and LDL-cholesterol: a controlled feeding trial. *European journal of clinical nutrition*, *64*(12), 1481-1487.
36. Lourenço-Lopes C, Garcia-Oliveira P, Carpena M, Fraga-Corral M, Jimenez-Lopez C, Pereira AG, Prieto MA, Simal-Gandara J. Scientific Approaches on Extraction, Purification and Stability for the Commercialization of Fucoxanthin Recovered from Brown Algae. *Foods*. 2020; 9(8):1113.

37. Matos PM, Mahoney B, Chan Y, Day DP, Cabral MMW, Martins CHG, Santos RA, Bastos JK, Page PCB, Heleno VCG. New Non-Toxic Semi-Synthetic Derivatives from Natural Diterpenes Displaying Anti-Tuberculosis Activity. *Molecules*. 2015; 20(10):18264-18278.

38. Miller KB, Eckberg JO, Decker EA, Marinangeli CPF. Role of Food Industry in Promoting Healthy and Sustainable Diets. *Nutrients*. 2021; 13(8):2740.

39. Millward DJ. Interactions between Growth of Muscle and Stature: Mechanisms Involved and Their Nutritional Sensitivity to Dietary Protein: The Protein-Stat Revisited. *Nutrients*. 2021; 13(3):729.

40. Multari, S., Stewart, D., & Russell, W. R. (2015). Potential of fava bean as future protein supply to partially replace meat intake in the human diet. *Comprehensive Reviews in Food Science and Food Safety*, *14*(5), 511-522.

41. Murdoch, J., Marsden, T., & Banks, J. (2000). Quality, nature, and embeddedness: Some theoretical considerations in the context of the food sector. *Economic geography*, *76*(2), 107-125.

42. Najmi A, Javed SA, Al Bratty M, Alhazmi HA. Modern Approaches in the Discovery and Development of Plant-Based Natural Products and Their Analogues as Potential Therapeutic Agents. *Molecules*. 2022; 27(2):349.

43. Ninkuu V, Zhang L, Yan J, Fu Z, Yang T, Zeng H. Biochemistry of Terpenes and Recent Advances in Plant Protection. *International Journal of Molecular Sciences*. 2021; 22(11):5710.

44. Normandin C, Boudreault P-L. Concise Large-Scale Synthesis of Tomatidine, A Potent Antibiotic Natural Product. *Molecules*. 2021; 26(19):6008.

45. Odhaib, K. J., Al-Hajjar, Q. N., & Alallawee, M. H. (2021). Incorporation of herbal plants in the diet of ruminants: effect on meat quality. *The Iraqi Journal of Veterinary Medicine*, *45*(1), 22-30.

46. Papotti B, Escolà-Gil JC, Julve J, Potì F, Zanotti I. Impact of Dietary Lipids on the Reverse Cholesterol Transport: What We Learned from Animal Studies. *Nutrients*. 2021; 13(8):2643.

47. Pop, O. L., Pop, C. R., Dufrechou, M., Vodnar, D. C., Socaci, S. A., Dulf, F. V., ... & Suharoschi, R. (2019). Edible films and coatings functionalization by probiotic incorporation: A review. *Polymers*, *12*(1), 12.

48. Proksch, P., Ebel, R., Edrada, R. A., Wray, V., & Steube, K. (2003). Bioactive natural products from marine invertebrates and associated fungi. *Sponges (porifera)*, 117-142.

49. Proshkina E, Plyusnin S, Babak T, Lashmanova E, Maganova F, Koval L, Platonova E, Shaposhnikov M, Moskalev A. Terpenoids as Potential Geroprotectors. *Antioxidants*. 2020; 9(6):529.

50. Raes, K., De Smet, S., & Demeyer, D. (2004). Effect of dietary fatty acids on incorporation of long chain polyunsaturated fatty acids and conjugated linoleic acid in lamb, beef and pork meat: a review. *Animal feed science and technology*, *113*(1-4), 199-221.

51. Rahaman MM, Azad MOK, Uddain J, Adnan M, Ali MC, Al-Mujahidy SMJ, Roni MZK, Rahman MS, Islam MJ, Rahman MH, Choi KY, Naznin MT. Microbial Quality Assessment and Efficacy of Low-Cost Disinfectants on Fresh Fruits and Vegetables Collected from Urban Areas of Dhaka, Bangladesh. *Foods*. 2021; 10(6):1325.

52. Rajas F, Gautier-Stein A, Mithieux G. Glucose-6 Phosphate, a Central Hub for Liver Carbohydrate Metabolism. *Metabolites*. 2019; 9(12):282.

53. Redondo-Blanco S, Fernández J, Gutiérrez-del-Río I, Villar CJ and Lombó F (2017) New Insights toward Colorectal Cancer Chemotherapy Using Natural Bioactive Compounds. *Front. Pharmacol*. 8:109.

54. Reis, F. S., Martins, A., Vasconcelos, M. H., Morales, P., & Ferreira, I. C. (2017). Functional foods based on extracts or compounds derived from mushrooms. *Trends in Food Science & Technology*, *66*, 48-62.

55. Ribeiro, J. S., Santos, M. J. M. C., Silva, L. K. R., Pereira, L. C. L., Santos, I. A., da Silva Lannes, S. C., & da Silva, M. V. (2019). Natural antioxidants used in meat products: A brief review. *Meat science*, *148*, 181-188.

56. Rochfort, S. (2005). Metabolomics reviewed: a new "omics" platform technology for systems biology and implications for natural products research. *Journal of natural products*, *68*(12), 1813-1820.

57. Saberi, B., Vuong, Q. V., Chockchaisawasdee, S., Golding, J. B., Scarlett, C. J., & Stathopoulos, C. E. (2017). Physical, barrier, and antioxidant properties of pea starch-guar gum biocomposite edible films by incorporation of natural plant extracts. *Food and Bioprocess Technology*, *10*(12), 2240-2250.

58. Shockley, M., & Dossey, A. T. (2014). Insects for human consumption. In *Mass production of beneficial organisms* (pp. 617-652). Academic Press.

59. Sharma, M., Usmani, Z., Gupta, V. K., & Bhat, R. (2021). Valorization of fruits and vegetable wastes and by-products to produce natural pigments. *Critical Reviews in Biotechnology*, *41*(4), 535-563.

60. Seid H, Rosenbaum M. Low Carbohydrate and Low-Fat Diets: What We Don't Know and Why We Should Know It. *Nutrients*. 2019; 11(11):2749.

61. Singh A, Dubey PK, Chaurasia R, Dubey RK, Pandey KK, Singh GS, Abhilash PC. Domesticating the Undomesticated for Global Food and Nutritional Security: Four Steps. *Agronomy*. 2019; 9(9):491.

62. Shipp, J., & Abdel-Aal, E. S. M. (2010). Food applications and physiological effects of anthocyanins as functional food ingredients. *The open food science journal*, *4*(1).

63. Stintzing, F. C., & Carle, R. (2004). Functional properties of anthocyanins and betalains in plants, food, and in human nutrition. *Trends in food science & technology*, *15*(1), 19-38.

64. Tang, D. Y. Y., Khoo, K. S., Chew, K. W., Tao, Y., Ho, S. H., & Show, P. L. (2020). Potential utilization of bioproducts from microalgae for the quality enhancement of natural products. *Bioresource technology*, *304*, 122997.

65. Thomford NE, Senthebane DA, Rowe A, Munro D, Seele P, Maroyi A, Dzobo K. Natural Products for Drug Discovery in the 21st Century: Innovations for Novel Drug Discovery. *International Journal of Molecular Sciences*. 2018; 19(6):1578

66. Turner, B. L., & Thompson, A. L. (2013). Beyond the Paleolithic prescription: incorporating diversity and flexibility in the study of human diet evolution. *Nutrition reviews*, *71*(8), 501-510.

67. Twaij BM, Hasan MN. Bioactive Secondary Metabolites from Plant Sources: Types, Synthesis, and Their Therapeutic Uses. *International Journal of Plant Biology*. 2022; 13(1):4-14.

68. Vanbergen, A. J., & Initiative, T. I. P. (2013). Threats to an ecosystem service: pressures on pollinators. *Frontiers in Ecology and the Environment*, *11*(5), 251-259.

69. Volek JS, Phinney SD, Krauss RM, Johnson RJ, Saslow LR, Gower B, Yancy WS Jr., King JC, Hecht FM, Teicholz N, Bistrian BR, Hamdy O. Alternative Dietary Patterns for Americans: Low-Carbohydrate Diets. *Nutrients*. 2021; 13(10):3299

70. Walker, R., Decker, E. A., & McClements, D. J. (2015). Development of food-grade nanoemulsions and emulsions for delivery of omega-3 fatty acids: Opportunities and obstacles in the food industry. *Food & function*, *6*(1), 41-54.

71. Yeshi K, Crayn D, Ritmejerytė E, Wangchuk P. Plant Secondary Metabolites Produced in Response to Abiotic Stresses Has Potential Application in Pharmaceutical Product Development. *Molecules*. 2022; 27(1):313.

72. Yousuf, B., Wu, S., & Siddiqui, M. W. (2021). Incorporating essential oils or compounds derived thereof into edible coatings: Effect on quality and shelf life of fresh/fresh-cut produce. *Trends in Food Science & Technology*, *108*, 245-257.

INDEX

M

N

O

P

Q

R

S